Community Power in Population Health Improvement

PROCEEDINGS OF A WORKSHOP

Anna Nicholson and Tamara Haag, *Rapporteurs*

Roundtable on Population Health Improvement

Board on Population Health and Public Health Practice

Health and Medicine Division

The National Academies of
SCIENCES • ENGINEERING • MEDICINE

THE NATIONAL ACADEMIES PRESS
Washington, DC
www.nap.edu

THE NATIONAL ACADEMIES PRESS   500 Fifth Street, NW   Washington, DC 20001

This activity was supported by contracts between the National Academy of Sciences and AAMC, Aetna Foundation, BlueCross BlueShield of North Carolina, Nemours, The Rippel Foundation, Robert Wood Johnson Foundation, The University of Texas at Austin, and Wake Forest Baptist Health/Stakeholder Health. Any opinions, findings, conclusions, or recommendations expressed in this publication do not necessarily reflect the views of any organization or agency that provided support for the project.

International Standard Book Number-13: 978-0-309-09349-1
International Standard Book Number-10: 0-309-09349-X
Digital Object Identifier: https://doi.org/10.17226/26306

Additional copies of this publication are available from the National Academies Press, 500 Fifth Street, NW, Keck 360, Washington, DC 20001; (800) 624-6242 or (202) 334-3313; http://www.nap.edu.

Copyright 2022 by the National Academy of Sciences. All rights reserved.

Printed in the United States of America

Suggested citation: National Academies of Sciences, Engineering, and Medicine. 2022. *Community power in population health improvement: Proceedings of a workshop.* Washington, DC: The National Academies Press. https://doi.org/10.17226/26306.

The National Academies of
SCIENCES · ENGINEERING · MEDICINE

The **National Academy of Sciences** was established in 1863 by an Act of Congress, signed by President Lincoln, as a private, nongovernmental institution to advise the nation on issues related to science and technology. Members are elected by their peers for outstanding contributions to research. Marcia McNutt is president.

The **National Academy of Engineering** was established in 1964 under the charter of the National Academy of Sciences to bring the practices of engineering to advising the nation. Members are elected by their peers for extraordinary contributions to engineering. John L. Anderson is president.

The **National Academy of Medicine** (formerly the Institute of Medicine) was established in 1970 under the charter of the National Academy of Sciences to advise the nation on medical and health issues. Members are elected by their peers for distinguished contributions to medicine and health. Victor J. Dzau is president.

The three Academies work together as the **National Academies of Sciences, Engineering, and Medicine** to provide independent, objective analysis and advice to the nation and conduct other activities to solve complex problems and inform public policy decisions. The National Academies also encourage education and research, recognize outstanding contributions to knowledge, and increase public understanding in matters of science, engineering, and medicine.

Learn more about the National Academies of Sciences, Engineering, and Medicine at **www.nationalacademies.org**.

The National Academies of
SCIENCES • ENGINEERING • MEDICINE

Consensus Study Reports published by the National Academies of Sciences, Engineering, and Medicine document the evidence-based consensus on the study's statement of task by an authoring committee of experts. Reports typically include findings, conclusions, and recommendations based on information gathered by the committee and the committee's deliberations. Each report has been subjected to a rigorous and independent peer-review process, and it represents the position of the National Academies on the statement of task.

Proceedings published by the National Academies of Sciences, Engineering, and Medicine chronicle the presentations and discussions at a workshop, symposium, or other event convened by the National Academies. The statements and opinions contained in proceedings are those of the participants and are not endorsed by other participants, the planning committee, or the National Academies.

For information about other products and activities of the National Academies, please visit www.nationalacademies.org/about/whatwedo.

PLANNING COMMITTEE ON COMMUNITY POWER IN POPULATION HEALTH IMPROVEMENT[1]

HANH CAO YU (*Chair*), Chief Learning Officer, The California Endowment, Oakland, CA
GARY R. GUNDERSON, Vice President, Faith Health, School of Divinity, Wake Forest University, Winston-Salem, NC
LOURDES J. RODRÍGUEZ, Senior Program Officer, St. David's Foundation, Austin, TX
ARVIND SINGHAL, Professor of Communication and Director of the Social Justice Initiative, The University of Texas at El Paso, El Paso, TX
ADITI VAIDYA, Senior Program Officer, Robert Wood Johnson Foundation, Princeton, NJ

---

[1] The National Academies of Sciences, Engineering, and Medicine's planning committees are solely responsible for organizing the workshop, identifying topics, and choosing speakers. The responsibility for the published Proceedings of a Workshop rests with the workshop rapporteurs and the institution.

ROUNDTABLE ON POPULATION HEALTH IMPROVEMENT[1]

SANNE MAGNAN (*Co-Chair through December 2020*), Senior Fellow, HealthPartners Institute, Emerald Isle, NC

JOSHUA M. SHARFSTEIN (*Co-Chair through December 2020*), Vice Dean for Public Health Practice and Community Engagement, Professor of the Practice, Johns Hopkins Bloomberg School of Public Health, Baltimore, MD

RAYMOND BAXTER (*Co-Chair from January 2021*), Trustee, Blue Shield of California Foundation, San Francisco, CA

KIRSTEN BIBBINS-DOMINGO (*Co-Chair from January 2021*), Professor and Chair of the Department of Epidemiology and Biostatistics; Lee Goldman, MD, Endowed Professor of Medicine; Vice Dean for Population Health and Health Equity, University of California, San Francisco, School of Medicine; San Francisco, CA

PHILIP M. ALBERTI, Senior Director, Health Equity Research and Policy, Association of American Medical Colleges, Washington, DC

DAWN ALLEY, Chief Strategy Officer, Center for Medicare & Medicaid Innovation, Washington, DC

JOHN AUERBACH, Executive Director, Trust for America's Health, Washington, DC

CATHY BAASE, Chair, Board of Directors, Michigan Health Improvement Alliance (MIHIA); Consultant for Health Strategy, The Dow Chemical Company, MIHIA, Saginaw, MI

DEBBIE I. CHANG, President and Chief Executive Officer, Blue Shield of California Foundation, San Francisco, CA

ALLISON GERTEL-ROSENBERG, Operational Vice President, National Policy and Practice Nemours, Washington, DC

MARC N. GOUREVITCH, Professor and Chair, Department of Population Health, New York University Grossman School of Medicine, New York, NY

GARTH GRAHAM, President, Aetna Foundation, Hartford, CT

MARGARET GUERIN-CALVERT, Senior Managing Director and President, Center for Healthcare, Economics and Policy, FTI Consulting, Washington, DC

---

[1] The National Academies of Sciences, Engineering, and Medicine's forums and roundtables do not issue, review, or approve individual documents. The responsibility for the published Proceedings of a Workshop rests with the workshop rapporteurs and the institution.

GARY R. GUNDERSON, Vice President, Faith Health, School of Divinity, Wake Forest University, Winston-Salem, NC
DORA HUGHES, Associate Research Professor of Health Policy and Management, Milken Institute School of Public Health, The George Washington University, Washington, DC
SHERI JOHNSON, Director, Population Health Institute; Acting Director, Robert Wood Johnson Foundation Culture of Health Prize; Associate Professor, Department of Population Health Sciences, School of Medicine and Public Health, University of Wisconsin–Madison, Madison, WI
WAYNE JONAS, Executive Director, Integrative Health Programs, H&S Ventures, Samueli Foundation, Alexandria, VA
ROBERT M. KAPLAN, Professor, Center for Advanced Study in the Behavioral Sciences, Stanford University, Stanford, CA
MICHELLE LARKIN, Associate Vice President and Associate Chief of Staff, Robert Wood Johnson Foundation, Princeton, NJ
MILTON LITTLE, President, United Way of Greater Atlanta, Atlanta, GA
PHYLLIS D. MEADOWS, Senior Fellow, Health Program, The Kresge Foundation, Troy, MI
BOBBY MILSTEIN, Director, ReThink Health, Morristown, NJ
JOSÉ T. MONTERO, Director, Center for State, Tribal, Local and Territorial Support; Deputy Director, Centers for Disease Control and Prevention, Atlanta, GA
VON NGUYEN, Senior Vice President and Chief Medical Officer, Blue Cross Blue Shield of North Carolina, Durham, NC
WILLIE OGLESBY, Interim Dean, College of Population Health, Jefferson University, Philadelphia, PA
JASON PURNELL, Vice President, Community Health Improvement, BJC HealthCare; Associate Professor, Brown School, Washington University in St. Louis, St. Louis, MO
LOURDES J. RODRÍGUEZ, Senior Program Officer, St. David's Foundation, Austin, TX
PAMELA RUSSO, Senior Program Officer, Robert Wood Johnson Foundation, Princeton, NJ
KOSALI SIMON, Herman B. Wells Endowed Professor, Associate Vice Provost for Health Sciences, Paul H. O'Neill School of Public and Environmental Affairs, Indiana University, Bloomington, IN
HANH CAO YU, Chief Learning Officer, The California Endowment, Oakland, CA

Health and Medicine Division Staff

ALINA BACIU, Roundtable Director
CARLA ALVARADO, Program Officer (*through January 2021*)
AYSHIA COLETRANE, Senior Program Assistant
HARIKA DYER, Research Assistant
ROSE M. MARTINEZ, Senior Director, Board on Population Health
    and Public Health Practice

Reviewers

This Proceedings of a Workshop was reviewed in draft form by individuals chosen for their diverse perspectives and technical expertise. The purpose of this independent review is to provide candid and critical comments that will assist the National Academies of Sciences, Engineering, and Medicine in making each published proceedings as sound as possible and to ensure that it meets the institutional standards for quality, objectivity, evidence, and responsiveness to the charge. The review comments and draft manuscript remain confidential to protect the integrity of the process.

We thank the following individuals for their review of this proceedings:

JASON PURNELL, BJC Healthcare; Washington University in St. Louis
IRENE YEN, University of California, Merced

Although the reviewers listed above provided many constructive comments and suggestions, they were not asked to endorse the content of the proceedings nor did they see the final draft before its release. The review of this proceedings was overseen by **BRUCE N. CALONGE,** The Colorado Trust. He was responsible for making certain that an independent examination of this proceedings was carried out in accordance with standards of the National Academies and that all review comments were carefully considered. Responsibility for the final content rests entirely with the rapporteurs and the National Academies.

We also thank staff member **ANA FERRERAS** for reading and providing helpful comments on this manuscript.

Contents

ACRONYMS AND ABBREVIATIONS		xvii
1	**INTRODUCTION**	1
	Workshop Objectives, 2	
	Organization of the Proceedings, 3	
2	**DARING TO LEAD**	7
	National Domestic Workers Alliance, 8	
	A Theory of Power to Achieve Change, 10	
	Radical Reimagining, 13	
	Discussion, 16	
3	**COMMUNITY POWER IN THE CONTEXT OF POPULATION HEALTH**	21
	Shifting Definitions of Power, 22	
	Addressing Power Dynamics in Health, 23	
	Personal Experiences in Power Building, 23	
	Addressing Internalized Devaluation, 25	
	Community-Building Influences, 26	
	Institutionalizing Power Building, 27	
	Objectivity and Relational Work, 29	
	Equality Improvement Conditions, 30	
	Progress in Power Building, 31	
	The Effect of Narrative on the COVID-19 Pandemic, 32	
	Values of People and Money, 34	

4	**COMMUNITY POWER: APPROACHES AND MODELS**	37

The Measure Care Model, 38
Healthy Richmond Collective-Building Policy Initiative, 41
The Positive Deviance Approach, 46
Discussion, 49

5	**FROM VISION TO ACTION: EFFECTIVE WAYS TO SUPPORT GRASSROOTS COMMUNITY POWER BUILDING**	53

Community Power-Building Ecosystem, 54
Partnerships Between Researchers and Community Groups, 56
Current Power-Building Strategies and Approaches, 60
Discussion, 68

6	**COMMUNITY-LED TRANSFORMATIONAL NARRATIVES**	73

Agency and Community Power, 74
The Power in Honoring Culture, 75
Go Austin/Vamos Austin Community Initiatives, 76
Church-Based Community Services, 77
Policy Advocacy for Health Equity, 78
Community-Centered Revitalization, 79
Discussion, 80

7	**AMPLIFYING THE EMPIRICAL BASE LINKING COMMUNITY POWER AND HEALTH EQUITY**	93

Personal Drive for Power Building, 94
Challenges and Tensions in the Exercise of Community
    Power: Practice Implications for Research, 95
The California Endowment: Building Healthy Communities, 99
Building Evidence for Power and Health: The BHC Initiative
    as a Learning Engine, 104
Community Power and Health Equity: The Memphis Model's
    Cardiac Disparity Case Study, 109
Community Empowerment and Health Equity: Practicing
    Community-Based Participatory Research in the Time
    of COVID-19, 113
Discussion, 116

APPENDIXES

A	References	123
B	Biosketches of Speakers, Moderators, and Planning Committee Members	127
C	Workshop Agenda	145
D	Readings and Resources	149

Boxes, Figures, and Table

BOXES

1-1   Statement of Task, 3
1-2   Workshop Highlights, 4
1-3   Definitions of Power Provided by Speakers, 5

2-1   Recognizing Oppression Within Oneself, 17

4-1   Healthy Richmond's Vision, Purpose, and Horizon Statements, 42

5-1   Robert Wood Johnson Foundation's Definition of Community Power, 55

FIGURES

2-1   The theory of power used by NDWA, 10

4-1   The MEASURE CARE model, 39

5-1   Domains of power in health, equity, and justice, 66
5-2   Approaches to cultural, political, economic, and transformative power building, 67

7-1 Power-building ecosystem, 102
7-2 Example of comparative interrupted time series design, 106

TABLE

7-1 Diverse Practices for Developing Community Power, 98

Acronyms and Abbreviations

AMI   acute myocardial infarction

BHC   Building Healthy Communities
BHCLB   Building Healthy Communities Long Beach
BVM   Black Voters Matter

CARE   community, advocacy, resilience, and evidence
CAUSE   Central Coast Alliance United for a Sustainable Economy
CBPR   community-based participatory research
CHN   Congregational Health Network
COVID-19   coronavirus disease 2019

GAVA   Go Austin/Vamos Austin

HIP   Human Impact Partners

ICSF   Iglesia Cristiana Sin Fronteras

JHU   Johns Hopkins University

LBF   Long Beach Forward
LGBTQ   lesbian, gay, bisexual, transexual, queer

MLH	Methodist Le Bonheur Healthcare
MSC	Movement Strategy Center
NDWA	National Domestic Workers Alliance
P3	possible, powerful, and probable
PICO	People Improving Communities through Organizing
RFF	Rockefeller Family Fund
RWJF	Robert Wood Johnson Foundation
SNF	Stavros Niarchos Foundation
TCE	The California Endowment
USC	University of Southern California
USC PERE	University of Southern California Program for Environmental and Regional Equity
UTEP	The University of Texas at El Paso
WFBH	Wake Forest Baptist Health

1

Introduction

To explore issues related to community-driven power-building efforts to improve population health, the virtual public workshop Community Power in Population Health Improvement convened on January 28 and 29, 2021, was hosted by the Roundtable on Population Health Improvement, Board of Population Health and Public Health Practice, at the National Academies of Sciences, Engineering, and Medicine. In the welcoming remarks, Kirsten Bibbins-Domingo, professor and chair of the Department of Epidemiology and Biostatistics and vice dean for population health and health equity at the University of California, San Francisco, highlighted that the roundtable recognizes that health and quality of life for all are shaped by interdependent, historical, and contemporary social, political, economic, environmental, genetic, behavioral, and health care factors. The roundtable seeks to provoke and catalyze urgently needed multisector community-engaged collaborative actions. The Community Power in Population Health Improvement workshop is premised on the belief that community leadership, voice, and power are essential drivers for successful population health efforts. In a relatively short amount of time, the field of population health has shifted the discussion of the role and potential of the community, moving from viewing community as a participant in population health efforts to acknowledging that the community is the rightful leader and driver of these efforts, said Bibbins-Domingo. She said:

> To lead, the community must exercise its power, as power is the driver to influence all social drivers of health. Power is wielded to shape those

factors that shape our lives. Although this realization is certainly not a new one and neither is the notion that community power shapes community well-being, the spaces where multisectoral lines of inquiry and conversation about power can take place are still limited.

The workshop was designed to feature advocates and subject-matter experts in community power-building efforts sharing their perspective, knowledge, and wisdom. Bibbins-Domingo noted that the roundtable aligns scientific research and evidence with lived experiences and narratives as fundamental and complementary tools for supporting community power, and she emphasized that the efforts carried out in and by communities are not new. What is new is the heightened and simultaneous attention that the community and its power are garnering from public and private sectors alike, which further spotlights the need for forums, roundtables, and additional spaces where discussions on power are held because collective power is built through relationships.

WORKSHOP OBJECTIVES

The workshop was organized in six sessions held over 2 days in a virtual format, featuring invited presentations and discussion that focused on the following:

- Understanding the underpinnings of community-led initiatives;
- Exploring power—its dynamics, manifestations, and narratives—as it pertains to the agency needed for communities to articulate their health and well-being needs and to act to address them;
- Exploring the approaches, elements, capacities, and ecosystems that support communities to lead their own efforts;
- Exploring the evidence base that links community power with systems of transformation and health equity outcomes;
- Listening and learning from examples of community-led population health efforts in action; and
- Communicating insights from entities supporting community-led efforts.

The Statement of Task to the planning committee is provided in Box 1-1. The workshop began with examples of effective power-building movements, then explored theoretical frameworks, models, and approaches for power building in the context of population health improvement, and concluded with practical applications and implications for the evaluation of linking community power with health equity outcomes. In accordance with the policies of the National Academies, the workshop did not

INTRODUCTION

> **BOX 1-1**
> **Statement of Task**
>
> A planning committee of the National Academies of Sciences, Engineering, and Medicine will organize a workshop that will explore community-led actions that improve population health. The workshop may feature presentations from speakers discussing the different components and dimensions of community-led action around different population health improvement topics such as education, transportation, environmental health, healthy eating, and active living, among others. A proceedings summarizing the presentations and discussions at the workshop will be prepared by a designated *rapporteur* in accordance with institutional guidelines.

attempt to establish any conclusions or develop recommendations about needs and future directions, focusing instead on issues identified by the speakers and workshop participants. In addition, the organizing committee's role was limited to planning the workshop. The proceedings of the presentations and discussions held at the workshop was prepared by designated rapporteurs in accordance with institutional guidelines.

ORGANIZATION OF THE PROCEEDINGS

The proceedings of this workshop is organized in seven chapters. Chapter 2, "Daring to Lead," highlights the initiatives and vision of leaders of two community-building organizations: the National Domestic Workers Alliance and the Black Voters Matter Fund. Chapter 3, "Community Power in the Context of Population Health," offers insights from two community organizers whose efforts are situated at the intersection of public health and civic engagement. Chapter 4, "Community Power: Approaches and Models," explores the practical applications of strategies for building community power. Chapter 5, "From Vision to Action: Effective Ways to Support Grassroots Community Power Building," examines approaches to community power building across fields, including perspectives from funders, advocates, and coalition builders. Chapter 6, "Community-Led Transformational Narratives," presents a variety of place-based initiatives, emphasizing the value of incorporating culture, history, and community knowledge in collaborative power-building efforts. Chapter 7, "Amplifying the Empirical Base Linking Community Power and Health Equity," explores the limitations of traditional research methodologies in evaluating power-building practices and examines the use of responsive assessment methods in this field. Brief highlights from

> **BOX 1-2**
> **Workshop Highlights**
>
> - Social determinants of health drive health outcomes, but power defines, drives, and shapes those social determinants. A shift is needed from a technocratic approach toward a more democratic approach to health that values people above all. (Brown, Ho, Iton, Poo, Speer)
> - Community narratives are a source of evidence that have the power to confront dominant narratives that normalize racism, white supremacy, misogyny, selfish individualism, and economic exploitation. (Brown, Carrillo, Ferdinand, Fernandes, Garza, Healey, Heller, James, Martinez, Poo, Styles)
> - A body of knowledge, expertise, and proven practices around community power building exists, generated by an array of practitioners and organizations dedicated to these efforts, and health professionals need to connect more fully with it. (Healey, Llanes Pulido)
> - Relationships are as important as technical solutions, and include institutional, personal, economic, and cross-cultural relationships. Relationships and their context are central to effective power-building practices. (Cutts, Fernandes, Garza, Gunderson, Han, James, Martinez, Parajón, Petit, Speer, Vaidya, Wright, Yu)
> - Community members hold solutions to issues in their communities and should determine power-building agendas, goals, and practices. Investing in community leaders, particularly youth and resident leaders, is critical. (Carrillo, Cutts, Fernandes, Frey, Garza, Gunderson, Han, Healey, Heller, Ho, James, Parajón, Petit, Singhal, Sostaita, Vaidya)
> - Currently, many institutions are failing society, making this a moment for transformation. (Brown, Heller, Ho, James, Poo)
> - An ecosystem of organizations with different capacities and capabilities is required to build power, organizing and base building, which are important for historically excluded populations to have power, agency, and voice. (James, Martinez, Vaidya)
> - Traditional research methods are not adequate to generate evidence of effective community-building practices, and responsive, immersive methods that capture variation are needed. (Cutts, Frey, Llanes Pulido, Styles, Wright)

the workshop are provided in Box 1-2, and an overview of the various definitions of power provided by different speakers is provided in Box 1-3. The references are in Appendix A; the biosketches of the speakers, moderators, and planning committee members are in Appendix B; the workshop agenda is in Appendix C; and recommended readings and resources are in Appendix D.

BOX 1-3
Definitions of Power Provided by Speakers

"The key word for this entire workshop is *power*, a word that is notorious for wobbly definitions and even outright discomfort in the classical, detached discourse of health science." (Milstein)

Power is "organizing people and resources, building long-term infrastructure to influence the political agenda." (Heller)

One definition is found in the "three faces of power"—a framework distinguishing among "power over," "power with," and "power to." (Milstein, referring to Healy and Hinson, 2005)

Another working definition of power is "organizing people and organizing money." (Healy)

What constitutes power relates to the tools available to effect societal change. (Healy)

"Community power is the ability of communities most impacted by structural inequities to develop, sustain, and grow an organized base of people who act together through democratic structures to set agendas, shift public discourse, influence decision makers, and cultivate ongoing relationships of mutual accountability to change systems and advance health equity." (Vaidya, quoting the Robert Wood Johnson Foundation definition)

Power is a multidimensional construct involving an ecosystem of strategies, processes, and partnerships. (Vaidya)

The domains of power that pertain to health equity are cultural power, political power, economic power, and, at the intersection of those three domains, integrated/transformative power. (James)

In Building Healthy Communities, "people power" evolved from "resident engagement" to "resident agency" to "power-building ecosystem." (Martinez)

2

Daring to Lead

CHAPTER HIGHLIGHTS

- Although the dominant approach to health is technocratic, health is better described as a democratic enterprise. (Iton)
- Power has many dimensions, including political, economic, narrative, and disruptive modeling. Avenues for the redistribution of power include policy change, culture change, innovation, and civic engagement. (Poo)
- Oppression of any group leads to the erosion of human value for all people. (Brown)
- New narratives can be created that affirm everyone's value, dignity, and well-being. Culture can be used to shift narratives and to help people connect with their power. (Brown, Poo)
- The disruption caused by the COVID-19 pandemic provides an opportunity for delivering real change. (Brown, Poo)

The first session of the workshop focused on the practical applications of power theory as used by leaders of movements for the rights of the domestic workforce and voter engagement. Participants discussed the effects of power on domestic workers and disenfranchised voters, as well as efforts to shift the power structure toward power sharing in a way that is centered on the values of respect and dignity for all human life. The session was moderated by Tony Iton, senior vice president of programs and partnerships at The California Endowment.

Iton noted that his organization is currently completing a 10-year Building Healthy Communities initiative, a "place-conscious" program that incorporates many of the factors discussed in this workshop such as changing the narrative and transforming communities most devastated by health inequities into places where all people have the opportunity to thrive. Although a technocratic approach to health is dominant in the system that trains most people who work in the field of health and health care, he suggested that health is better described as a democratic enterprise. "In a democratic enterprise what matters is power and a sense of belonging and ultimately for folks to come together to work on root cause conditions," Iton stated, offering the shorthand of *ABC* to represent this dynamic: *A* is for *agency*, *B* is for *belonging*, and *C* is for *changing conditions*. These factors are at play in the community-led initiatives featured in this workshop.

NATIONAL DOMESTIC WORKERS ALLIANCE

Ai-jen Poo, co-founder and executive director at the National Domestic Workers Alliance (NDWA), described the conditions faced by domestic workers in the United States and efforts underway to build power within this workforce. NDWA advocates for quality work, dignity, and fairness for the growing number of workers who clean homes and care for individuals, the majority of whom are immigrants and women of color.[1] Founded in 2007, NDWA has partnered with more than 60 local affiliates and more than 200,000 members to pass domestic worker bills of rights in nine states and to bring minimum wage protections to over 2 million home care workers.

Scope of Issues Facing Domestic Workers

Poo provided an overview of the domestic worker population in the United States. Noting that domestic workers have been on the "front lines of every dimension of the COVID-19 [coronovirus disease 2019] crisis," she said there are currently approximately 2.5 million individuals working for more than 5 million employers in more than 5 million workplaces nationwide. These occupations include nannies who provide childcare, house cleaners who maintain order and sanitation in homes, and home care workers who care for the aging and support people with disabilities to live independently in their homes and remain connected in their communities. She described domestic labor as "the work that makes all other

---

[1] More information about the National Domestic Workers Alliance is available at https://www.domesticworkers.org (accessed February 8, 2021).

work possible," noting that this labor has always been essential. Yet, she added, it is some of the most uncertain and undervalued work in the American economy today, as reflected in the rights and benefits lacking in most domestic jobs, such as contracts, retirement benefits, health care, consistent hours, the right to unionize, a minimum wage, overtime pay, and weekends off.

Providing a historical context, Poo outlined factors contributing to the lack of security in domestic work. Traditionally performed by women, an underlying assumption that women will continue to provide these services—regardless of pay—has long influenced domestic working conditions. Furthermore, professional domestic work has historically been associated with women of color, as enslaved Black women served as some of the first domestic workers in the United States. Since then, Black, Indigenous, immigrant, Brown, and Asian Pacific Islander women have composed the majority of the domestic labor workforce. Since the 1930s, the historical ways in which race and gender have shaped both this nation and this workforce have been codified into laws that systematically excluded domestic workers from basic labor rights.[2] The result is an entrenched view that domestic labor is not real work, as demonstrated by the application of the term *help* to this field, she contended. Additionally, the nature of domestic work presents unique structural challenges to improving conditions and raising standards for this workforce. For instance, no registry exists to track the locations in which domestic workers are employed. Driving through any neighborhood, it is impossible to identify which houses are workplaces. The hidden and isolated nature of domestic labor poses barriers to identifying and connecting workers in the millions of residential workplaces across the United States.

The mission of NDWA is to support domestic workers and enable them to live and work with dignity. Poo noted this mission builds on the work of generations of Black women who organized to improve conditions and build power for this workforce. In spite of this history, challenges persist. Domestic labor is associated with poverty wages; coupled with the lack of access to health care or a safety net, these factors contribute to high levels of job insecurity. She highlighted the effect of the COVID-19 pandemic, which has been devastating for both the domestic workforce and for the people who depend on these workers. As baby boomers age and people live longer, the expanding aging population in the United States will increase the demand for home care workers. Whereas the growth of all U.S. jobs is expected to increase by 6.5 percent from 2014 to 2024, the growth in personal care aides and home health aides is anticipated to

---

[2] See, for example, the description of the Fair Labor Standards Act omission of domestic workers at https://www.dol.gov/agencies/whd/direct-care/faq (accessed June 2, 2021).

expand by 25.9 percent and 38.1 percent, respectively, during the same time period (Hogan and Roberts, 2015). Poo emphasized that these jobs, which cannot be outsourced or automated, will make up a large share of jobs in the future, yet the current average annual income for a home care worker is just $17,000 per year. These poverty wages signify "This workforce that we count on to care for us cannot take care of their own families," Poo stated.

A THEORY OF POWER TO ACHIEVE CHANGE

The theory underpinning NDWA's work is that centering the domestic worker community allows for power building along multiple dimensions, resulting in a transformation of the quality of domestic jobs and the future for this workforce, Poo explained. She then described the four dimensions of power: political, narrative, economic, and disruptive/modeling (see Figure 2-1).

Poo defined political power as both the ability to change policy and the ability to determine who makes policy. Narrative power is the capacity to explain and justify the legitimacy of power structures in place and maintain the status quo. Economic power is the ability to direct capital and shape markets. Disruptive and modeling power leverages the ability to build compelling models and disrupt the status quo to convey the urgency of needed change. Models for the future can demonstrate that alternatives to the status quo are both possible and scalable, she noted. The approaches used by NDWA to achieve needed changes involve

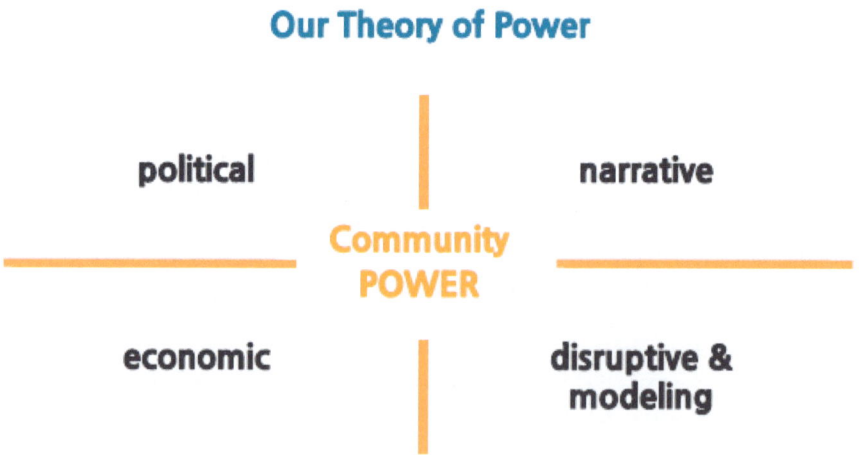

FIGURE 2-1 The theory of power used by NDWA.
SOURCE: Presentation of Ai-jen Poo, January 28, 2021.

organizing people around civic engagement, innovation, policy, and culture. For example, this work can take the form of mobilizing voters and advocating for policy change. It also includes changing the media narrative and cultural norms around the domestic workforce and industry. Furthermore, building innovative products, especially in the technology space, can improve conditions for this workforce, Poo added.

Policy Change

Outlining a number of successes that NDWA has achieved, Poo described the organization's foundational work that took place in New York City. In the late 1990s, organizers brought community members together in immigrant community centers and church basements. This work eventually led to the launch of a statewide campaign to establish the first Domestic Workers' Bill of Rights in the United States.[3] This campaign involved thousands of domestic workers in communities across New York State in a 7-year effort and resulted in the passage of the Bill of Rights in 2010. This achievement inspired domestic workers to organize at the community level across the country. In the 11 years since, domestic worker legislation has passed in nine states: California, Connecticut, Hawaii, Illinois, Massachusetts, Nevada, New Mexico, New York, and Oregon. Furthermore, legislation has passed in Philadelphia and Seattle that pushes the envelope further to bring more power and voice to the domestic workforce, Poo continued. Seattle created the first-ever Domestic Workers Standards Board,[4] which brings all industry stakeholders together to define the norms and standards that shape the future of domestic work in that city. In Philadelphia, NDWA won the right to portable paid time off for domestic workers in the United States,[5] the first time such a right has been established in this country. The city is currently in the midst of implementing this policy, she added.

Poo noted that these legislative achievements scale up to the national level. Built upon community-level work, a National Domestic Workers Bill of Rights was introduced into the Senate by Kamala Harris before she vacated her Senate seat to become the U.S. vice president.[6] NDWA has launched a coalition effort of every constituency with a stake in creating

---

[3] More information about New York State's Domestic Workers' Bill of Rights is available at https://labor.ny.gov/legal/domestic-workers-bill-of-rights.shtm (accessed March 3, 2021).

[4] More information about Seattle's Domestic Workers Standards Board is available at https://www.seattle.gov/domestic-workers-standards-board (accessed March 3, 2021).

[5] Refers to benefits that follow workers between jobs.

[6] More information about the National Domestic Workers Bill of Rights is available at https://www.nytimes.com/2019/07/14/opinion/harris-jayapal-domestic-workers.html (accessed February 9, 2021).

a strong care economy, including older adults, people with disabilities, and family caregivers (Poo, 2019). Additionally, NDWA is advocating for universal family care, a social insurance fund that would help people pay for childcare, paid leave, and long-term care (Poo and Veghte, 2019). Poo explained that this concept would enable people to access care for their families while they are working outside the home, while simultaneously investing enough money into the system to enable every job in the care economy to provide a living wage, benefits, and real economic security.

Culture Change and Innovation

To access the narrative dimension of power, NDWA partners with artists to tell the stories of the domestic workforce. An example is the film *Roma* (2018), in which the protagonist is a domestic worker, and around which NDWA built a campaign for culture change in partnership with the film's producers.[7] Poo said this type of storytelling can shape both popular narrative and culture, demonstrating that domestic workers are the "unsung heroes in our lives" and are the "protagonists not only in their own lives and in our homes, but in our future."

The NDWA innovation lab has created a portable benefits platform called "Alia" that allows domestic workers to gain access to benefits, such as paid time off and various insurance products, for the first time.[8] Poo explained that during the COVID-19 pandemic, NDWA has been able to leverage this platform to deliver emergency cash assistance to more than 50,000 domestic workers who were negatively affected by the pandemic but did not have access to any type of federal relief.

Civic Engagement

Poo asserted that all these efforts have shaped the public narrative, ultimately resulting in real-life improvements for domestic workers. For example, during his presidential campaign, Joe Biden announced a $775 billion plan to invest in the U.S. care economy to support working families and the caregiving workforce as part of his economic recovery strategy for responding to the COVID-19 pandemic (Miller et al., 2020). Needed change "begins and ends in community," she emphasized. NDWA hosts meetings of democratically elected councils of workers from local communities around the country. These councils collaborate to define needed

---

[7] NDWA developed a case study describing this work. See https://www.domesticworkers.org/wp-content/uploads/2021/05/Roma-Case-Study.pdf (accessed July 2, 2021).

[8] More information about Alia is available at https://www.ndwalabs.org/alia (accessed February 15, 2021).

standards, determine what it means to have respect and recognition, and establish what it looks like to have health and safety in communities. Next, the councils work together to discern how to make this vision real. These efforts are fueled by a belief that community-driven solutions and community-rooted power building are the future, said Poo. The future of health, of care, and of American democracy all depend upon elevating the people who have been long failed by our systems to the forefront of this process. She explained that this is not only for their benefit, but for "the sake of a healthy, multiracial democracy that can sustain and support us across generations." Poo concluded that if communities who have not had power within American democracy are given that power, it will benefit all people and lead to "the future we deserve."

RADICAL REIMAGINING

LaTosha Brown, co-founder of the Black Voters Matter (BVM) Fund, a power-building, Southern-based, civic education organization, spoke about the need for a vision of an equitable world that is centered on human value. An organizer, philanthropic consultant, activist, and singer–songwriter, Brown is the principal owner of TruthSpeaks Consulting LLC, a philanthropy advisory consulting firm, the project director of Grantmakers for Southern Progress, and the co-founder of BVM Capacity Building Institute.

Envisioning a World Without Racism

Although models and strategies for organizing are needed, Brown's remarks focused on "a greater conversation that is not happening." She asked participants to close their eyes and consider the question: what would America look like without racism? Regardless of whether the setting is an Ivy League school, a corporate room, or a community center, people find this question difficult to answer because racism has become normalized and deeply integrated into how people interact with and perceive one another. While many people say they want to address and end racism, this cannot happen without first being able to envision it. Thus, in order to bring a nonracist, nonsexist nation into being, the first step is "radically reimagining" what the systems of a country that focuses on human value and that opposes the oppression of human life would look like. Brown remarked that while conversations about policy, programs, and approaches are common, innovation in how we see ourselves in human relationships is rarely discussed. Questioning how we see human value is often missing from discussions on change.

Erosion of Human Value

Brown remarked that a challenging component of racism is that people have accepted that there are some positive attributes to racism, particularly in the white community. She continued that while racism does provide some level of privilege to those in the "primary race that is lifted up in white supremacy," an "erosion of human value across the board" is taking place. Racism erodes human value for all people, including those who are privileged by the system. Brown contended that the reason the United States does not have universal health care is not simply because millions of Americans profess not to want it. Rather, it is rooted in the efforts of the Freedmen's Bureau to expand health care to newly released enslaved Africans during the period of Reconstruction. A cadre of white political actors opposed this move, establishing a value that persists to this day. Currently, it is not only Black people who do not have access to health care, but also white, Asian, and Indigenous people. Brown asserted that an erosion of thinking around human value, rooted in an institution of slavery that some thought would only affect Black people, is responsible for the millions of Americans of all races who do not have access to health care.

"We've got to have an honest conversation of how racism destroys our belief around human value for *all* human life," Brown emphasized. She said:

> The moment that you open up your mind [to the idea] that there are some people that are more worthy than other people, the moment you open up your mind on that, it actually erodes your belief in human value. The moment that we become okay that there are children locked in cages because they have a different color passport or that there are some people who are called "aliens," as if they are from another planet, the moment that we open our mind to that theory, we have accepted that there is some erosion of our belief of human value.[9]

She continued by saying that too often conversation around policy is driven by outcomes while neglecting process. A narrow focus solely on a specific outcome can be detrimental, she noted, giving the example of a school that increased from poor to high performance within 2 years. Expecting to find that structural changes and a shift in expectations enabled this school to turn performance around so quickly, Brown instead

---

[9] In referencing "children locked in cages," Brown is referring to the federal family separation policy instituted in 2018 in which child immigrants entering the United States were separated from their parents and detained under the supervision of the U.S. Department of Health and Human Services.

discovered a policy had been enacted that enabled the school to remove low-performing students from the school entirely. This practice gave the appearance that the school's performance had increased, but in actuality, they were strategically removing students to improve the overall average. Brown described this as an example of how data can be tailored to support any desired narrative. Thus, rather than merely being data driven, Brown maintained that a love for humanity should be at the core of all change efforts.

Vision and Agency in Political Power

Brown reflected on a world in which each and every sector was driven by the love of humanity: "How will we interact with each other? What would the field of science look like? What would the field of medicine look like? What would government and politics look like?" During the U.S. presidential election on November 3, 2020, and the two U.S. Senate runoff elections on January 5, 2021, the majority of votes in the state of Georgia were cast for Democratic candidates for the first time in 2 decades. In dissecting this political shift, many people look for specific actions that were taken. Brown said nothing new was added to the "get-out-the-vote" model that has been used in the past and across the country. Rather, the transformative element was that instead of centering a candidate or a political party, BVM and other voting advocates reminded people that they have agency, power, and the right to shape everything that governs them in their lives. Brown noted that when a program centers itself around human value, this creates a shift that leads to transformation.

Seldom in politics is the goal of human development the focus, Brown said. She remarked that her "goal has never been democracy ... [for] as a nation, we have killed people under the name of democracy, we have made and extracted wealth from people in the name of democracy, as if democracy is actually greater than the people." Rather, she suggested that democracy is a means to an end—not an end in itself—and it seems like the best way forward is working toward the goal of recentering the notion of love of humanity. Brown explained that she roots a love of humanity in her politics and in the model of organizations she creates, refusing to reduce people to data points or desired outcomes.

Brown concluded by encouraging the audience to radically reimagine what a nation without racism could look like and to use innovative thinking to shape the systems needed to realize this vision. Not only will this involve changing external systems, but it will also require reordering people around a central notion of human value.

DISCUSSION

Facilitating Power Building

Racism, sexism, and anti-immigrant sentiment shape both the perceptions of the constituents within a community and how policy makers view those constituents, Iton commented. Given that stigma, devaluation, and dehumanization may be internalized by the members of communities being organized, Iton asked how to approach working with people whose experience of oppression and its associated trauma may have limited the ways in which they view their own power. Poo suggested that this work should focus on creating the context for people to connect to their agency and power, saying:

> That is really what we do all day, every day, is to figure out how we, through community, through connection, and through action, actually create the context for people to understand just how powerful they are and just how much unique value they offer to our communities, to the work that they do, and to our country as a whole.

Poo added that this created sense of community and connection extends beyond power to encompass a sense of self, of belonging, and of collective confidence. In turn, this shared power can be used to change the conditions of people's lives.

Brown added that real change centers the notion of human value. The effects of programs and strategies will be limited to the culture within which they are operating. When a society organizes itself around the idea that some human life does not have value, the result will be homelessness, exploitation, lack of health care, hunger, and an environment destroyed by climate change. In a value system that has eroded, Brown asserted, "the only thing that really matters is success, winning, and money, and not human life." She noted that all people, herself included, are subject to devaluing others. She reflected on an experience in which she recognized that oppression lives within herself (see Box 2-1).

Approaches to Shifting Narratives

Iton asked what strategies can be used to shift mindsets by amplifying and diffusing new narratives to the greater public. Furthermore, he asked how narratives have been employed to support civic engagement, culture change, innovation, and policy. Poo said the first step in challenging and replacing dominant narratives is to analyze them. For example, dominant narratives that devalue human life see some forms of work as "real work" and other forms as "less than." Similarly, some people are

> **BOX 2-1**
> **Recognizing Oppression Within Oneself**
>
> Once I was at Gladys Knight's Chicken and Waffles in Atlanta, Georgia. I was on a diet, and this was going to be my one "cheat meal." As I was walking in, a homeless man was sitting outside eating food someone had given him. I went inside and ate my cheat meal. Of course, if you know about a "cheat meal," you know I didn't want to eat it all and wanted to save some to eat later. As I was going outside, the same man I greeted on my way in asked me for my food. In the culture of my family and in the deep South, if someone asks for food, I must oblige, no matter who it is. If you ask me for food, I have to feed you. It doesn't matter what I'm doing, I have to stop and feed you. Because of my family culture, when this man asked for food, I had to oblige. As I begrudgingly gave him my food, I said, "You probably eat better than me." He looked at me and said, "What, I shouldn't?"
>
> It messed me up. I couldn't sleep that night. It bothered me at first, and my first reaction was defensiveness. I thought, "Why would you say that to me? I'm a social justice activist. I fight for social justice." But the truth of the matter is, when I said to him, "you probably eat better than me," embedded in that was the belief that because I worked hard every day that I should be eating better than him because he was a homeless man. Now, I would never say that. But that belief lived in me. And in that moment, that belief was revealed to me. Since that time, I'm constantly recognizing that I am trained in a particular context, and I ask myself, "How does oppression live in me?"
>
> SOURCE: Adapted from Brown presentation, January 28, 2021.

seen as more human than others. These dominant narratives about who works and who matters must be uncovered. In beginning to replace them, Poo recalled Brown's exercise of envisioning what society would look like without those narratives. She asserted that all people should challenge themselves to envision what replacement narratives—that is, those that affirm everyone's value, dignity, and wellness—might look like. Lastly, people should put those new narratives into the environment via day-to-day activities, the media, and popular culture, building momentum around the narratives that should shape the future rather than holding on to narratives that perpetuate the status quo.

Brown stated that "culture will eat strategy for breakfast." No matter how excellent the plans, they must be aligned with the culture of the community to take hold. Culture should not be ignored within the health care space, Brown advised. Rather, culture can be used to communicate, to affirm, and to help people access power in their communities. For many people, the reason they like to travel is to see other communities operating in their authentic voice of culture, Brown explained. She described how when she travels to Jamaica, she does not want to hear the Southern accent and eat the grits and bacon that she finds in her hometown of Atlanta. Rather, she wants to experience the local foods—like oxtails and fresh fish with the eyes still in them—and hear the local patois. When she travels to France, she is intrigued with the way people sway as they walk and sit outside at cafes. Being in another culture "almost forces us to recognize the value in someone else," Brown stated, adding that "culture should not just be a commodity in the entertainment industry;" its socially affirming quality should be used as an organizing tool.

Often, the approach used to counter a narrative actually continues to center the narrative that those efforts are intending to shift, Brown contended. She suggested that instead, new narratives should focus on the people living in communities and be designed in a way that encourages people and awakens their sense of imagination. She noted that many people are predisposed to enjoy the powerful gift of imagination, as demonstrated by the popularity of Disney World and cartoons. Too often, hard science is exclusively relied upon while disregarding the importance of culture, Brown remarked, adding that culture "is a science that has been created and perfected over thousands of years by a particular people based on a particular environment, based on a particular similar experience." The power of culture should not be overlooked, she concluded. Poo added that data, arguments, and research are overly relied upon when attempting to create change. However, the attitude that society can research its way toward equality ignores that people are complex and emotional beings. In trying to effect change, it is not only the factual, rational minds of humans that must be considered, but also their emotional landscape. Reaching people as humans on an emotional level is foundational to achieving the change that we want and need, said Poo.

Harnessing Opportunities for Disruption

Iton noted the considerable opposition community organizers face, citing the legislature and government apparatus in Georgia that appears to be involved in voter suppression and the series of institutions that have treated the domestic workforce as expendable, disposable, and largely irrelevant in the policy space. Given the influence of these institutions and institutional norms, Iton asked how disruptive power can be leveraged in health institutions and in the concept of how health is created.

Poo replied that the present moment is an optimal time to leverage power, given that the COVID-19 pandemic has wrought such significant disruptions to the ways people live, work, and care across the country, and these present an opportunity to set new norms, narratives, and behaviors. Furthermore, the pandemic has spotlighted essential workers. Whereas before COVID-19 there was an epidemic of low-wage work—with millions of working Americans unable to afford rent, food, and necessities—the pandemic has revealed that not only is this work dignified, it is also essential to safety and survival. The disruptions caused by the pandemic have created an opportunity for a collective effort to impart real change and cement these new narratives into policy, behaviors, norms, and practices. Poo described the health sector as the "tip of the spear" for recovery from the pandemic, which can set the pace of change in the fight for racial and gender equity. "You do not have to figure out how to create [disruption]. The question is how to pull the thread toward equity and justice," she said.

Brown emphasized that institutions are created by people: just as people can change, so too can institutions, and "when people change and their values change, the institutional values will change." Outcomes have been prioritized over purpose, she asserted, resulting in an inappropriate focus on programs and processes over people themselves. Regarding the opportunity afforded by the COVID-19 pandemic, Brown recalled that her grandfather, who lived to the age of 104 years, used to say, "Until the pain of staying the same becomes greater than the pain to change, people will never change." In that sense, she said, the discomfort we feel can be seen as a gift that helps to reorder our thinking around how to move forward. Science can be used for more than merely advancing health outcomes; it can be used to provide factual evidence that when people are treated better, all people benefit, she added.

The present moment is well situated for reflection around the institutional changes that are needed, Brown suggested. At times, people become attached to institutions that have outlived their need and no longer serve a function. In such cases, people may be more attached to the institution than the outcome. Brown said she looks forward to the day when the Black Lives Matter movement is no longer needed—but for that day to arrive, the work must be centered around a vision of equality.

3

Community Power in the Context of Population Health

CHAPTER HIGHLIGHTS

- Power can be seen as organizing people and resources, building long-term infrastructure to influence the political agenda, and helping people make meaning of events. (Heller)
- Building alliances between organizations and with legislatures creates effective political and legislative tools. (Healey)
- Centering community voices in research and advocacy is a component of building power and addressing oppression. (Healey, Heller)
- Dominant narratives have led to inequities and must be replaced with a new, unified, collective narrative that addresses issues of white supremacy and individualism. (Healey)
- Power building requires infrastructure built around the mission of changing society. Institutions must invest resources into a broader mission beyond internal efforts. (Healey)
- The response to the COVID-19 pandemic was hampered by decades of underfunding of public health fueled by dominant narratives—grounded in individualism—that the government is incompetent, and the free market can solve collective problems. (Heller)

The second session of the workshop featured a discussion of current community power-building efforts and focus areas for future work. The discussion featured Richard Healey, founder and senior advisor at the

Grassroots Policy Project and chair of the board of the Commonwealth Foundation for Inclusive Democracy, and Jonathan Heller, senior health equity fellow at the University of Wisconsin–Madison's Population Health Institute and co-founder of Human Impact Partners (HIP).[1] The discussion was moderated by Bobby Milstein, director of systems strategy at ReThink Health.[2]

Milstein remarked that the workshop was designed to deepen understanding of how to enlist greater numbers of people in community-building work and help them to establish their own roles in building power. Although there are currently great opportunities to change systems and cement new narratives, he acknowledged that those efforts could feel daunting owing to a lack of buy-in. Sharing expertise is helpful in determining how the difficult but healthy work of affirming human value and agency can be incorporated into norms and routines. Milstein noted that collectively, Healey and Heller have 70 years of experience working at the interface of population health and civic life—an intersection where people's power to shape a common world, as well as their own lives and livelihoods, comes into focus.

SHIFTING DEFINITIONS OF POWER

"The key word for this entire workshop is *power*, a word that is notorious for wobbly definitions and even outright discomfort in the classical, detached discourse of health science," said Milstein. However, it is possible to examine the pragmatic experience of building power to identify its features. Referencing Healey's "three faces of power"—a framework for strengthening movement infrastructure—Milstein asked about the framework's distinctions between "power over," "power with," and "power to" (Healy and Hinson, 2005). He also asked for examples of manifestations of these aspects of power. Healey described community-organizing efforts in Chicago, Illinois, in the early 1970s. He already had years of experience in activism at that point and was drawn to the community-organizing efforts taking place in the city. To be successful, this work involved the organization of both people and money. Thus, their working definition of power

---

[1] More information about Grassroots Policy Project is available at https://grassrootspolicy.org (accessed February 17, 2021). More information about the Commonwealth Foundation for Inclusive Democracy is available at https://commonfound.org (accessed February 17, 2021). More information about the University of Wisconsin–Madison's Population Health Institute is available at https://uwphi.pophealth.wisc.edu (accessed February 17, 2021). More information about Human Impact Partners is available at https://humanimpact.org (accessed February 17, 2021).

[2] More information about ReThink Health is available at https://www.rethinkhealth.org (accessed February 17, 2021).

became "organizing people and organizing money." At that time, efforts were constrained to the local level. Often, the work took the form of four or five staff members working to get community members elected to local office and better positioned to advocate for improved conditions for their neighborhoods. While organizers were aware of structural racism and social determinants of health, those concepts were not discussed explicitly at the time. Only recently has the power of narrative—the focus of the previous session—become embraced, he added. Healy reflected that as recently as a decade ago, people threatened to kick him out of community-organizing meetings when he talked about power as narrative, ideology, and storytelling, because it was not viewed as a practical approach.

Healey remarked that although there is no single definition of power, his interest is in expanding the notion of power in ways that enable community groups to expand the tools at their disposal. Over the past 10 years, narrative has been incorporated into the definition of power. The dominant perspective in the past was that people and money were organized locally, but the power of building major, durable alliances has also emerged as a component of the working definition of power. He added that the notion of what constitutes power relates to the tools available to effect societal change.

ADDRESSING POWER DYNAMICS IN HEALTH

Milstein asked how health professionals can create space to consider power dynamics and building power. Heller noted that health inequities received little attention in public health discourse 15 years ago, but more recently, the topic has developed into a prominent narrative theme. These health inequities are largely caused by inequities in the social determinants of health, such as housing, voting access, and income, he noted. Across these areas, people of color with low incomes are generally the most affected, mostly as a result of power imbalances and oppression. Thus, if health equity is to be advanced, power imbalances must be addressed. He added that the field of public health can address issues that communities care about by centering their voices and helping them build power to achieve their goals. This work can involve partnering with community-organizing groups, such as the National Domestic Workers Alliance (NDWA), he continued.

PERSONAL EXPERIENCES IN POWER BUILDING

Milstein asked about the circumstances that led the panelists, both applied methodologists, to a career path focusing on power building. Healey said he is the third generation of a family of activists who escaped

Hungary. When he was an epidemiologist for the State of Massachusetts, he looked at the environmental causes of chronic diseases. This involved going to cities such as Woburn and Canton to explore possible associations between increased cancer rates and environmental hazards.[3] This work led him to think more deeply about the role of power, after state senators and corporations attacked him and the community for discussing environmental causes of cancer because of fears that it would drive down property values. Healy noted that he was often unsuccessful in those attempts to center people, not property values. However, over time, he and others in this field, including colleagues at this workshop, have slowly developed tools of power. Community groups are no longer isolated in advocating for themselves and in fighting forces much larger than themselves. Instead, statewide alliances are developing ever-more sophisticated political and legislative tools. Milstein reflected that behind any environmental, housing, or health crisis, there is a power crisis, and that the people determining the circumstances leading to these crises may not value—and may even actively resist—the idea of making space for everyone to thrive.

Heller commented that his own history of approaching health problems through examination of power dimensions is more recent. Initially, he used his Ph.D. in biophysics in a biotechnology career. However, he was drawn to the health field after witnessing the suffering caused by malaria during his service in the Peace Corps. He came to see that biotechnology was not the best strategy to address issues such as malaria, and he did not feel he was living in alignment with his values. Thus, he shifted to public health, wanting to bring a data lens to creating solutions. Heller recalled, "[I was] naively thinking that if I just did reports, like health impact assessments, and brought data to decision makers, they would change their minds. Lo and behold, more data does not actually change things." Fifteen years ago he started to understand this when he volunteered with environmental justice advocates who were organizing in West Oakland, California. A low-income housing development for seniors was proposed next to the freeways by the port, and the organizers were concerned about the seniors' exposure to pollution and noise. During a 3-month process, the organizers held five meetings in which community members discussed the issues surrounding the housing development. Input from those meetings was used to draft a 10-page letter regarding the potential health impacts of locating low-income senior housing next to the freeway and port. This letter, containing both data and stories from the community, was sent to the developers, only to be ignored. However,

---

[3] Healey and colleagues investigated an increase in the occurrence of childhood leukemia from 1969 to 1979 in Woburn, Massachusetts (Cutler et al., 1986).

a group member had a relationship with a planning commissioner, who happened to be involved in the nurses' union, and the member sent the letter to that commissioner. A commission meeting was held around the development, and the planning commission asked the developers to work with the community group. "It was not necessarily the data that changed anything," Heller contended, it was the relationships and power, paired with the data, that resulted in the developers changing their plans and ushering in other changes in Oakland. Reading "The Three Faces of Power" (Healy and Hinson, 2005) helped Heller understand that power was fundamental to all the issues activists address, including housing, incarceration, immigration, and that a shift in power was necessary for change. Health and community organizing fit in that framework, he concluded.

ADDRESSING INTERNALIZED DEVALUATION

Milstein highlighted the key role of power in issues of equity and justice, as demonstrated when the initial efforts of the community organizers were ignored by the developers during Heller's experience in West Oakland. He contended that the tendency to ignore the needs of devalued people must be met with efforts to gain dignity and respect for devalued groups, just as NDWA and the Black Voters Matter (BVM) Fund are doing. He emphasized that the first step in any kind of move to improve health has to be rooted in the dignity and inclusion of people. He asked for examples of people who were ignored or oppressed yet managed to gain the dignity they deserve in the eyes of those overlooking or devaluing them.

Healey remarked that he first recognized this needed shift toward dignity while advocating for a living wage for hotel service staff. He witnessed that many of these low-paid workers had internalized a low sense of self-worth in response to "the dominant, neoliberal[4] narrative that you are worth what you are paid." Thus, the starting point must be helping people understand that all humans have equal value, regardless of wealth or fame. Identifying allies who validate that sense of self-worth, such as ministers and city councilors, is part of the process. Healey noted that public health professionals are well positioned to serve as validators. The dominant narrative in the United States has long been that those not earning much money are at fault for their circumstances and, in turn, they are blamed for not getting more education or training. In contrast, he suggested, the narrative that should be strengthened is that working people are worthy of the right to earn a living wage and that their children

---

[4] See https://plato.stanford.edu/entries/neoliberalism for a definition of neoliberalism.

are worthy of receiving good childcare. Healey said the struggle with the political conditioning and the internalized dominant narrative is "a crucial piece of this puzzle."

This approach aligns with HIP's work and focuses on the concerns of community members Heller described. Instead of coming into communities and telling residents why they should be concerned about an issue, HIP listens to community members about the issues that are important to them. Partnering with community-organizing groups, HIP assists with the issues the community members have prioritized. For example, if members are concerned about housing, HIP works with organizers on rent or other housing-related issues. While avoiding forcing a health perspective on community members, HIP pulls from the considerable research available around housing and health, a research area that has been growing in the past 20 years. Heller noted that the scientific perspective on research can be limiting; input from community members is valuable data that should be incorporated. For instance, in conversations with communities in Minnesota around access to education, critical race theory was raised, alerting HIP that the research literature was limited in terms of adequately describing the experiences members were sharing. By bringing the community voice alongside the published research and government data, HIP simultaneously filled a gap in the research and demonstrated to community members that their real-life experience is valuable and needed. After HIP issues a report, they work with the community to convey the contents of the report to city councils, state legislatures, or other advocacy avenues. Heller emphasized that the entire process is focused on validating community concerns, bringing the voices of the community together, and helping community members build their power to tackle issues affecting their lives.

COMMUNITY-BUILDING INFLUENCES

Milstein commented that lifting up human dignity and helping people change the circumstances of their lives requires a shift or evolution in how knowledge is pursued. He asked the panelists about influences on their practice of science centered around human dignity and the narrative of people's agency. Healey replied that he was influenced by activists and radicals in his family, and also by the work of Stuart Hall, a Jamaican sociologist, activist, and theorist of narrative and cultural strategies. Providing a public health example of such strategies, Healey said the dominant (cultural) narrative of individualism is tied to white supremacy and ignores collective struggles. Within this narrative, focus is placed on promoting oneself while competing with everyone else and treating health as a commodity that individuals seek out, while dismissing socialized medicine as an impractical framework. Over decades, this narrative has led to the devaluation of public health and other public agencies, making health something that can be attained if one can afford it. In turn, Healey asserted, poor people, and particularly people of color, are excluded from access to health care. The health conditions on reservations for Indigenous people in the United States reflect this exclusion. Healey suggested that a new collective narrative is needed for examining public versus private health at the intersection of race and individualism. Furthermore, community groups, public health groups, and trade unions should seek to ensure that the narratives of their respective organizations are addressing questions of white supremacy and individualism. He added that public health is particularly well positioned for this work.

Heller shared the insights about power he gained from Healey's framework. Initially he was dismissive about ideas of power until "The Three Faces of Power" provided him with an understanding of how the pieces fit together, Heller described. He described Jamaican-British sociologist Stuart Hall as a key influence on the topics of narrative and cultural strategies. Community organizers such as Deepak Bhargava from Community Change,[5] Doran Schrantz from ISAIAH,[6] and others were instrumental in helping Heller shift from a perspective of hard sciences to a focus on relationships and organizations. In applying public health ideas to community organization, he built on the foundation laid by such leaders as Tony Iton, senior vice president of programs and partnerships at The California Endowment (TCE),[7] Jeanne Ayers of VoteSafe Public Health,[8] and others who have long been advocating for health equity. Heller said he melded the ideas learned from these experts with community-organizing principles to inform the way he analyzes the world and approaches his work at HIP and the University of Wisconsin.

INSTITUTIONALIZING POWER BUILDING

Milstein thanked Heller for sharing that he had previously dismissed the role of power in public health, noting that many people do not fully understand the meaning or gravity of power. He asked what actions could be taken to help institutions incorporate the value of working from

---

[5] More information about Community Change is available at https://communitychange.org (accessed March 19, 2021).

[6] More information about ISAIAH is available at https://isaiahmn.org (accessed March 19, 2021).

[7] More information about The California Endowment is available at https://www.calendow.org (accessed March 19, 2021).

[8] More information about VoteSafe Public Health is available at https://www.astho.org/votesafepublichealth (accessed March 19, 2021).

an understanding of power so that these efforts are not dependent on individual personal transformation. Milstein said methodologies such as community-engaged research and health impact assessments have a role, and Healey has referred to the pivotal role of organizers in mediating relationships necessary for instigating change. How can the importance of power be brought to bear on institutional priorities, Milstein asked. Healey replied that an organization's understanding of how it can build its power and its working definition of power inform where that organization will invest its resources. An organization that invests all its resources in building its own internal work may find this to be effective, Healey noted, but he has focused his work on putting resources into deeper, more powerful alliances—in a sense, organizing other organizations. For example, he has worked on multiple projects linking community organizers with local health departments. This enterprise is challenging, considering the varied missions and internal cultures community organizers and state health departments have. These organizations are constrained by the political bodies they report to, and their immediate mission is different than that of community organizations. Healey said his work has been developing approaches to advance beyond these challenges to the deeper issues of human value and dignity addressed in the previous session. This involves allocating resources into relationship-building efforts between different types of organizations to build a larger institution. Building an infrastructure requires uniting various parts, each carrying out different tasks, around the mission of changing society. The operative question then becomes how an institution decides to put resources into a broader mission, Healey suggested.

Heller added that this is the type of work HIP began 3 years previously, through funding from TCE, to bring together health departments and community-organizing groups to work collaboratively. A HIP pilot program identified five health departments in California, then matched each county health department with a local community-organizing group. The county health department agreed to help the community-organizing group build power by working on the group's focus issue. The community-organizing group agreed to work with the health department and bring a health lens to organizing work. Building relationships was a crucial step that took place over the first year, Heller explained. As these organizations have different missions and their approaches vary from one another, building relationships was fundamental to the process. The pilot began with a 2-day meeting in Oakland, California.

Heller noted that after the first day of programming, participants from the Santa Barbara Health Department and its community partner, Central

Coast Alliance United for a Sustainable Economy (CAUSE),[9] went out to dinner together. The experience of sharing food initiated a relationship between the organizations, a shift that was apparent to Heller the next day as the groups ate breakfast together. This relationship enabled the organizations to collaborate effectively on an issue of focus for CAUSE's members: conditions for farm workers. Their workers did not have access to toilets, which is a basic, fundamental health issue. Using the power of the Santa Barbara Health Department, the partnership was able to elevate the importance of this issue in the county over the course of a year. Furthermore, Heller has seen ripple effects of these efforts. For example, organizing groups working with farm communities have reported that many undocumented workers lack trust in their health departments and therefore have uncertainty regarding recommendations related to the COVID-19 pandemic. In contrast, the relationships established in Santa Barbara have built trust; Heller was hopeful that this trust has translated to mitigating the impact of COVID-19 on the undocumented farm-worker community in that area.

Healey commented that the decision to have dinner together is contingent on having the resources available to do so. Community-organizing groups are perpetually resource constrained, both financially and in staffing. Resources provided by TCE enabled Heller and HIP to allocate time to facilitating relationships. Not only can philanthropy enable organizers to spend time with the community members they are serving, but it also enables organizers to work with legislatures, forming connections and highlighting the value of the efforts being made. Such relationships can be protective in establishing defenders should an organization make controversial moves toward change. When community organizations, trade unions, health departments, and legislatures work together, it shields people from attack, enabling them to work beyond their usual comfort level without fear of being fired. Creating this type of space and security requires resources, which gives philanthropy an important role to play in community organizing, Healey concluded. Milstein remarked that it can seem like resources are the constraint, but it is possible to view resources as abundant if they are invested into building wider relationships.

OBJECTIVITY AND RELATIONAL WORK

Given the norm of detached objectivity in health science, Milstein asked how a commitment to this type of relational work can be approached alongside objectivity and scientific neutrality. Healey replied that science

---

[9] More information about CAUSE is available at https://causenow.org (accessed March 11, 2021).

tells us that racism and white supremacy have had a destructive effect on people of color and on white people in the United States. "That is good science ... not bias," he commented. Structural income inequality and social determinants of health are objective facts. He suggested that people who are interested in improving human health should leverage the scientific knowledge that is available to advocate for changes to the political, social, and economic structures that perpetuate health inequality, such as racial segregation and mass incarceration. Healey remarked that this can be done "objectively and passionately, because science is on our side."

Heller remarked that this question of objectivity is one he has considered at length. When he came into this work, he thought data alone could solve problems in public health. He quickly realized that this is not possible and came to understand that the concept of objectivity in this context is false. Everyone has values, including scientists, and these values influence the research questions asked, the answers received, how results are presented, and which research gets funded. Given the extent to which values and beliefs shape the research process, the idea that science is purely objective is a false narrative, he asserted. However, public health departments can take advantage of that narrative by validating community concerns, giving them scientific language, and including them in scientific publications. He added that the community-organizing groups he works with are often viewed as political and biased. When he and his team conduct health impact assessments, collecting data through focus groups and scientific methodology, they can report data in a way that is more palatable to decision makers than messaging from community-organizing groups. Thus, the perception that public health is objective can be used to present data in more effective ways to certain groups that might otherwise dismiss it, he said.

Healey highlighted the need for careful consideration about what is construed as objective knowledge, because it is not limited to expert knowledge or results of the scientific process—"tacit knowledge or experiential knowledge is absolutely crucial." People with lived experience have knowledge that is critical to incorporate.

EQUALITY IMPROVEMENT CONDITIONS

Milstein echoed Iton's statement, made earlier in the workshop, that although health is often seen as a technocratic enterprise it would be better framed as a democratic enterprise. He noted that "equality improvement" has become a watchword in health care, and he reflected on the circumstances that are needed to engage greater numbers of people in a joint, orchestrated enterprise that establishes conditions in which everyone can thrive. He asked the panelists to discuss ways to mobilize enough engagement in such an enterprise to ensure that the people affected are determining the opportunities for action—rather than funders or organizations—if the field shifts away from its current reliance on experts and institutions to do this work alone.

Healey responded that those in power are often wary when people organize, because democracy can be a threat to the status quo. Once people experience organizing around an issue, they may expand to other issues. He said the founders of the United States were afraid of democracy and thereby created a relatively weak government, as a true democracy could result in property being shared, white supremacy being overturned, and people speaking for themselves and working together as they realize their larger self-interests. Continued efforts to disenfranchise people stem from fear of democracy, he added. Isolated people "often feel like they have no power, and in some sense, they do not." When individuals are brought into larger structures by groups such as the BVM Fund and NDWA, they often discover that it makes sense to be engaged in the public sphere. As an isolated individual, it can be difficult to see the difference one can make; in being part of a larger group, the value of engagement and participation becomes more evident. Healey suggested that continued investment in "down-home organizing" could help local people to understand their stake in an issue and feel more confident that they will get a return on their participation in efforts to achieve change.

PROGRESS IN POWER BUILDING

The infrastructure that enables people to engage in organizing is grounded in being relational and engaged, rather than observational and technocratic, Milstein commented. He asked about progress toward facilitating the power shift necessary to center people's voices and create an infrastructure that can make this practice routine. Healey remarked on the substantial progress in this direction since he began this work in the 1970s in Chicago. At that time, modern community organizing was in its infancy and was competitive, with groups attacking one another for resources and encouraging funders to stop funding other groups. The idea that community organizations could work together was inconceivable, he said. In the years since, national networks of community organizations have formed and ties have been established among community organizations, trade unions, and religious and civic institutions. However, in spite of this progress, the infrastructure remains insufficient, Healey emphasized. Only in the past few years have community organizations become meaningfully involved in electoral politics, for example. The accomplishments of LaTosha Brown, co-founder of the BVM Fund; Stacey Abrams; and other Black women in Georgia illustrate the shift from the antipolitical notions of community organizers of the 1970s to the recent emphasis on entering electoral politics as a legitimate arena of power.[10] Healey described this as an exciting change but noted that much work remains to be done.

Healy also remarked on the current lack of a common narrative—around race, gender, capitalist institutions, individualism, and white supremacy; there is no shared narrative across the institutions of public health, community organizing, and organizing around workers, housing, low-income people, and the unemployed. A unified message is needed to effectively communicate across institutions and across the country. Healey said that fragments of this narrative are commonly known, with white supremacy being a major issue and dog-eat-dog capitalist competition playing a role, but work needs to be done to accomplish change in bigger terms.

Heller agreed on the need for a new narrative and new infrastructure to further the participation of the groups listed above and others. Collaborating with Ai-jen Poo, co-founder and executive director at NDWA, and others through the Always Essential campaign, he is currently facilitating an alternative type of worker organization tailored to nonunion worker groups that have formed around issues related to the COVID-19 pandemic and the essential worker framework. Although this is an example of certain infrastructure pieces coming together, those elements also need to be strengthened, Heller said. In addition to the contributions of community-organizing groups, the health sector also has a large role to play in this infrastructure, as do governments and other institutions. Public health agencies and hospitals have relationships with other institutions and with individuals that they can bring to this growing infrastructure. Organizers are excited about working with public health agencies because of their relationships with planning departments, public works departments, and other governmental agencies. In giving community-organizing groups access to these governmental relationships, public health agencies can support power building through establishing power-sharing infrastructure, added Heller.

---

[10] Stacey Abrams and LaTosha Brown led efforts to address voter suppression and engage Black voters. Record turnouts of Black voters have been credited for democratic wins in Georgia in the November 3, 2020, presidential election and two U.S. senate runoff elections on January 5, 2021.

THE EFFECT OF NARRATIVE ON THE COVID-19 PANDEMIC

Milstein raised the issue of the various social dynamics at play in the COVID-19 pandemic, which have underscored the extent to which population health and community health are underfunded relative to health care. The social context and interdependency of our lives are highlighted during times of crisis and often ignored in ordinary times, he said. Organizational efforts toward dignity, inclusion, and conditions for all people to thrive are going largely unnoticed by institutions, with hospitals and public health partners unaware of community groups that have been working in their own neighborhoods for decades. He added that targeted disinformation is tearing at people's sense of belonging, connection, and dignity. Bearing these social dynamics in mind, Milstein asked whether there is a way to spring forward from the current crisis into a renewal of civic life.

Heller remarked that many of the dominant narratives have led to dynamics present in the current crisis. These include the narrative that the government is incapable of doing anything right, that the free market is able to solve our collective problems, and that the government should thus be decreased in size. This line of thinking has led to underfunding public health for decades, resulting in the complete lack of preparedness for the current public health crisis, he maintained. Another dominant narrative is "pull yourself up by your bootstraps" individualism. COVID-19 is a collective issue, intertwining the health of individuals with one another; still, the response has been grounded in individualism. For instance, people have been told to stay at home and take care of themselves. Collective responses, such as paid sick days, are not being used. Heller stated the individualistic narratives need to change, and noted that messages such as "we are all in this together" are emerging, but are not yet universally embraced. The crisis of the pandemic, Heller asserted, has revealed the degree to which the United States is ill prepared, that corporations do not have all the answers, and that a collective response in the form of government is needed. The government has failed many people for centuries, but the collective response to the COVID-19 pandemic has underscored that failure in a dramatic way. Echoing Healey's earlier call for a shared narrative, Heller said a compelling and consolidated narrative is needed in order to prepare for the next public health crisis.

Healey offered an example of the work that remains to be done from California, a state that appeared to have a strong health system, with good hospitals and quality of health care. However, over the past 20 years, hospitals have been decreasing bed numbers to save money. Profitability, resources, and disinvestment have been taken for granted, even in a non-profit setting, with profitability serving as the dominant narrative. During the COVID-19 pandemic, the lack of redundancy has translated into a lack of buffers and resiliency because of a failure to appropriately prepare for long-tail probability events. He said that in the short term, allowing for redundancy does not seem smart or efficient. However, COVID-19 has shown that tethering health to profitability can be hugely detrimental for individuals. Referencing Brown's earlier talk about centering human value in decision making, Healey emphasized the need to move away from the narrative of profitability of health and determine other types of criteria for health decisions.

VALUES OF PEOPLE AND MONEY

Milstein referenced the recent release of the Surgeon General's *Community Health and Economic Prosperity* report, which established that healthy communities are needed to prosper economically, and an inclusive economy is needed for everyone to be healthy.[11] Without both community health and economic prosperity in place, society can spiral into adversity; when they work in tandem, opportunities arise for both to grow simultaneously. Although the language of the political left and of the right can be further explored, Milstein remarked that neither Healy nor Heller is suggesting these issues stem solely from a red–blue partisan divide. He also noted a recent *Harvard Business Review* article that showed that 9 out of 10 Americans would be willing to receive less pay in order to do more meaningful work (Achor et al., 2018). He asked whether this desire to be a part of something bigger than one's private paycheck and family resources is a signal that unifying American society is possible.

Healey replied that when he talks with people in small groups about issues that matter to them (e.g., the meaningfulness of work), the distinction between right versus left politics tends to evaporate. In holding such discussions around the country—including in rural, predominantly white areas—he has heard white people talk about health care in terms of not wanting the wages cut of people caring for family members and not wanting profit to be considered above whether somebody lives or dies. Healey stated that there is something "wrong with thinking about profit and loss in health care" and noted that health has a special role in framing these issues in human terms, rather than in political terms.

Heller noted that personally, he chose to take a decrease in income

---

[11] The report is available at https://www.hhs.gov/sites/default/files/chep-sgr-full-report.pdf (accessed February 17, 2021).

in exchange for more meaningful work. Biotechnology pays far more than the nonprofit world, but Heller said making the change was the best decision of his life. It gave meaning to his life, made him a happier person overall, and was the right thing to do, he reflected. More broadly, Heller said he sees the future of work in the United States changing—for example, with increased automation and companies like Amazon surveilling their workers,[12] there is potential for harm until the narrative changes around what is allowed. Heller suggested that the fundamental question is which is more valued: people or solely profits. A shift will have to take place to create the kind of world in which everyone can thrive, Heller said, and it is that shift that community organizers are driving toward.

---

[12] See, for example, https://www.openmarketsinstitute.org/publications/eyes-everywhere-amazons-surveillance-infrastructure-and-revitalizing-worker-power (accessed February 21, 2021).

4

Community Power: Approaches and Models

CHAPTER HIGHLIGHTS

- Traditional data collection and research methods have betrayed the communities of Black and Indigenous people, and people of color, and these traditional methods must be disrupted with the development of equitable data tools. (Styles)
- Strategies for effective power building include creating safe spaces for participation, cultivating strategic relationships, creating paths for different levels of community engagement, leveraging the inherent strength of residents, and equipping community members with an understanding of how policy and systems work. (Garza)
- The positive deviance approach is based on the fundamental premise that in any community that faces a complex social problem, there exist people who have already solved the problem while facing higher odds and with no extra resources. (Singhal)

The third session of the workshop showcased existing models for community-based learning and evaluation, each grounded in principles of power building and in asset-based, people-centered frameworks. The session featured presentations on using quantitative and qualitative data in antiracist work, community planning to incorporate resident voices in development decisions, and the positive deviance community-based approach to solving public health problems. Lourdes Rodríguez, senior program officer at St. David's Foundation, moderated the session.

THE MEASURE CARE MODEL

Meme Styles, founder and president at MEASURE, discussed the historical gap in equitable data tools and the work being conducted to fill it. MEASURE is a nonprofit, social enterprise in Austin, Texas, that uses an antiracist revenue model to provide free data support to Black- and Brown-led organizations. To provide this free data support, MEASURE asks white-led corporations, organizations, and universities to pay the full rate for services.[1] The organization uses the CARE (community, advocacy, resilience, and evidence) model in working with community groups to build power and use data in generating solutions and advocating for change.

Filling an Equitable Data Tools Gap

Styles described that racism data and research is complex, and it can be perverse and opportunistic. Having the potential to perpetuate racism, this research can treat people of color as "petri dishes," by analyzing them and applying methodological frameworks to explain their experiences without ever asking them about those experiences. In an effort to address the lack of accessibility of equitable data tools, MEASURE provides free data support to Black- and Brown-led organizations. Styles explained their team is comprised of Black and Brown female data activists; the team includes doctors, lawyers, scientists, mothers, college students, and people recently released from incarceration. Adding lived experience to quantitative data, the group takes research to action by mobilizing the community to generate solutions.

The Black, Indigenous, and people-of-color communities have been betrayed by traditional academia, data collection, and research, said Styles. To disrupt the traditional research methodologies created in an environment of structural racism, MEASURE has developed evaluation tools to combine qualitative and quantitative data about complex social problems affecting people of color. The organization's evaluation tools have gone through an extensive community-led process to ensure that MEASURE authentically represents the people with whom it works. Styles added that the group routinely evaluates its tools and processes to make sure the work it conducts is antiracist. MEASURE's antiracist revenue model provides services at a full rate to white-led groups and organizations

---

[1] More information about MEASURE is available at https://wemeasure.org (accessed February 21, 2021).

with the economic means to afford data services, while providing Black- and Brown-led organizations services at no charge; this model has been appealing to other organizations in Austin, Texas, and beyond.

The CARE Model

Styles emphasized that until an equitable framework is built into public administration models, tools, and health systems, the risk of the continual cycle of racism remains within the largest American social services and institutions. Thus, MEASURE was intentional in developing equitable tools that use data to create change. The result is the CARE model, a system she described as "game changing" (see Figure 4-1). This model breaks the community mobilization process into four components: community, advocacy, resilience, and evidence. Organizations and institutions can use the CARE model with any issue they are partnering with communities to address, whether it be health, criminalization, or voting rights. Increasing meaningful community engagement while minimizing potential trauma or harm to that community, the CARE model is based on the following four guiding principles: (1) community is involved from the beginning; (2) advocacy within communities is used to address disparities, resulting in power building; (3) solutions are generated that strengthen community resilience; and (4) data and evidence inform decision making.

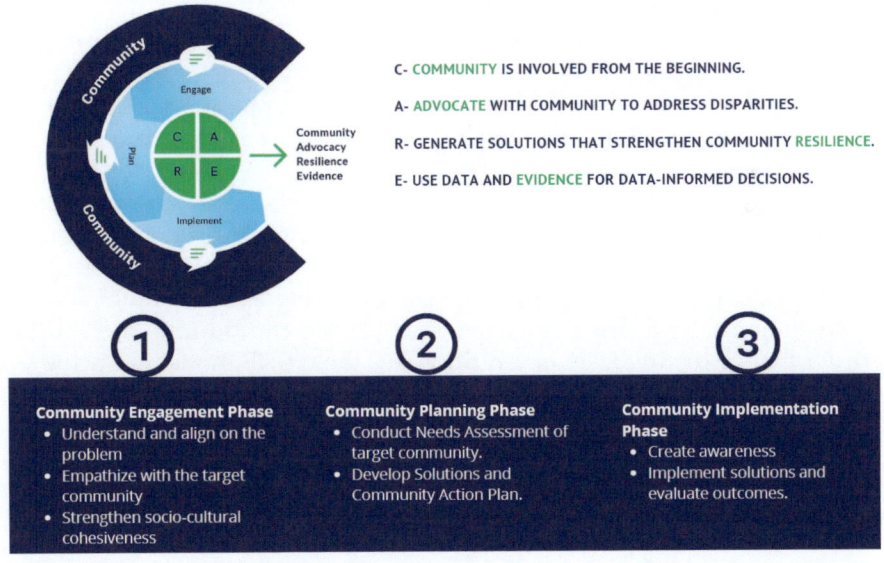

FIGURE 4-1 The MEASURE CARE model.
SOURCE: Styles presentation, January 28, 2021.

Methodology of the CARE Model

Styles provided an overview of the methodology of the CARE model, which requires 3 months to complete. Each time MEASURE is invited to work with an organization, it strives to initiate a robust partnership. The work begins with a community engagement phase, during which understanding and alignment on the issue is developed, empathy for the target community is cultivated, and sociocultural cohesion is strengthened. This process involves a thorough understanding of what has taken place to perpetuate injustice in the community around the issue at hand. The second phase is community planning, which involves a needs assessment of the target community, solution development, and a community action plan. The final phase of community implementation includes raising awareness, implementing solutions, and evaluating outcomes. CARE teams are formed to identify community impact metrics for tracking progress on outcomes and outputs. These data are then used to assess the group's theory of change.

Effect of the CARE Model in Central Texas

Styles described the effect of the CARE model implemented in central Texas. The Innocence Initiative is an award-winning program that has trained more than 700 attorneys to protect Black girls from adultification bias.[2,3] This effort led to the creation of a community-created policy brief that is informing new laws in Texas, along with the distribution of "15,500 community-created comic books about Black girl magic." The program has launched a mentorship program that matches Black girls with Black women, in addition to providing them with food, monthly cash stipends, and access to two Black women psychologists who are part of the program's team.

When the COVID-19 pandemic hit, MEASURE was able to rapidly convene its community around the proven CARE model, Styles explained. It conducted a needs assessment, collecting more than 900 responses from people of color regarding how they were affected by the pandemic. This assessment helped drive resources back to the community and quickly drive change during a crisis. Additionally, the CARE model has achieved legislative impact through the formation of "increasing equity" circles,

---

[2] More information about the Innocence Initiative is available at https://wemeasure.org/wp-content/uploads/2020/12/MEASURE_-The-Innocence-Initiative-2020-School-Local-Policy-Brief-1.pdf (accessed February 22, 2021).

[3] Adultification bias "is the perception of Black children as less innocent and more adultlike than their white peers" (Epstein et al., 2017).

which are groups that work to change legislation affecting their communities. Styles gave the example of a small town that created a new law to form the first equity commission. She noted that an unexpected outcome of using the CARE model has been the launch of new nonprofits led by people of color.

Next Steps for the CARE Model

Styles said MEASURE is grappling with the best ways to increase impact, including fundraising efforts. In 2020, the organization offered a college course on data activism at Huston-Tillotson University, a local historically Black college. Prioritizing equity and research, the course was developed with the goal of creating a pipeline of Black and Brown researchers. The pilot class during fall semester of 2020 was successful and was offered again with a second cohort the following semester. Styles added that MEASURE is working to bring this course to Texas State University in the fall of 2021. Additionally, MEASURE is training CARE model facilitators who will work with organizations serving people of color. The goal is to recruit 20 new certified MEASURE educators to use the organization's tools with other groups, Styles added. This would expand the capacity of the group, which was able to provide 1,239 hours of free data support to Black- and Brown-led organizations in 2020. MEASURE is also working to affect the research community, she said. To help disrupt traditional research methods, the organization is training researchers at major institutions on how to the use the CARE model and other activist-created tools.

HEALTHY RICHMOND COLLECTIVE-BUILDING POLICY INITIATIVE

Roxanne Carrillo Garza, senior director at Healthy Richmond,[4] works with resident leaders, community-based organizations, base builders, and systems leaders to develop collective policy advocacy strategies to improve health, safety, school and neighborhood environments, and economic development opportunities. She outlined her organization's vision statements and its strategies for power building in economic, educational, and health equity.

Healthy Richmond is a collective-building policy initiative in the San Francisco Bay area launched by The California Endowment 10 years ago, Garza explained. The group approaches policy advocacy by partnering

---

[4] More information about Healthy Richmond is available at https://healthyrichmond.net (accessed February 23, 3021).

with resident leaders, organizations, and system allies to work toward health equity and racial justice. In 2019, the group held several racial equity dialogues in order to update its vision, purpose, and horizon statements to guide race equity work over the following 3 years (see Box 4-1). Garza noted that these statements include explicit language regarding race equity and eliminating anti-Black racism, thus positioning the organization to meet the moment as the events of 2020 unfolded.[5]

Building Power for Education Equity

To address education equity, Healthy Richmond has supported parent and student leaders in advocating within the local school district. Garza stated that in 2014, the school district underestimated parents' ability to understand the complexities of California legislation, called the Local Control Funding Formula, that then-Governor Jerry Brown put into place to help close equity gaps for specific student populations. She noted that over the next 7 years, parent and student leadership demonstrated that they were indeed able to understand the complexities of the legislation. They also engaged in the following activities:

BOX 4-1
Healthy Richmond's Vision, Purpose, and Horizon Statements

Vision statement: Healthy Richmond envisions a transformed community where resident leaders (youth and adults), community-based organizations, and system leaders work together to shift power and create equity within and across education, economy, health care, and safe communities to increase race equity and eliminate racism.

Purpose statement: To empower and mobilize organizational and resident leadership most affected by race inequity and anti-Blackness to transform and make radical changes to address racism in our community and system in order to build power and reallocate resources.

Horizon statement for race equity: Demonstration of collective impact and power building for public systems change in Richmond that is rooted in healing and eliminating anti-Black racism and centers resident leaders and young people.

SOURCES: Garza presentation, January 28, 2021; https://healthyrichmond.net/about-hr (accessed March 8, 2021).

---

[5] On May 25, 2020, George Floyd was killed during an arrest by a policeman who knelt on his neck for more than 8 minutes. Widely shared video footage of Floyd's death led to worldwide protests calling for racial justice and the end of police brutality.

- Researching the data on the district's academic performance;
- Creating the We Are the Experts curriculum to train peers on how to be civically engaged;
- Consulting with regional experts on school-based, social-emotional health models;
- Looking at the legal implications of the district's decision-making processes at the local level; and
- Developing annual policy platforms and presenting these to the superintendent and school board.

The group has built power and a voice within the school district, backing policies on positive school climate and a resolution on African American achievement that successfully passed. Current efforts focus on creating a racial equity community oversight council, which would allow parents to work in partnership with the school board to define what racial equity in the district looks like. Thus far, the school board has not been supportive of this step, Garza noted.

Strategies for Power Building in Education

In Healthy Richmond's education equity efforts, Garza said that five key strategies have emerged. The first strategy is to create safe spaces for participation. She explained that encouraging community members to become actively engaged in policy discussions and decisions requires more than inviting them to meetings, particularly when the community members have historically been excluded. Real engagement calls for thoughtful attention to community cultures and contexts in creating spaces for discussion that feel safe and welcoming. This involves taking time to break down policy jargon, encouraging questions and discussion, and having bilingual staff in place to enable participants to speak in their native languages.

The second strategy is to invest in "reach" to ensure broad participation. Healthy Richmond developed training that includes a focus on aligning messages and creating common scripts, which enables clear, accurate, consistent information to be shared during the recruitment engagement process. Garza said partners need to recognize how difficult it can be for community members to participate in workshops or trainings, given their work schedules and family demands. This informs the third strategy, creating paths for community engagement at different levels. Not every resident will be able or willing to go to a board meeting, Garza noted. Offering an array of paths for engagement of varying degrees of intensity allows for greater participation. These paths can include workshops, town halls, school district advisory committee meetings, and intensive organizing trainings. By affording parents and students a range of opportunities to participate, they can choose to engage in ways that feel comfortable to them and meet their needs.

Fourth, cultivating strategic relationships and community is key to power building, said Garza. Supporting relationship building between parents, advocacy organizations, and school leaders provides parents with direct connections to the decision makers and organizations that can help them achieve their goals. Strong relationships across families are also needed to create a sense of solidarity across cultures, thus rooting advocacy efforts in a strong sense of unity. Garza described this step as critical to the work. Lastly, allocating time to reflect and celebrate is the fifth strategy for power building, because community celebrations can help residents remain motivated and hopeful. Taking time to learn from any missteps and reflect on opportunities to conduct future campaigns in different ways fosters resilience in facing the persistent challenges presented by these systems, she added.

Building Power for Economic Justice

Using an approach built on the foundation of community organizing, Healthy Richmond worked with North Richmond resident leaders to create a quality-of-life plan. Garza explained that the plan was intended to highlight residents' priorities and aspirations for their community to inform future development. Healthy Richmond worked with resident leaders to (1) facilitate a deeper understanding of their leadership and change-making potential, (2) use their voices to hold stakeholders accountable, and (3) exercise real power. A team of ten resident leaders conducted an analysis of the strengths, weaknesses, opportunities, and threats within their neighborhood. Engaging more than 200 residents, leaders conducted resident interviews and held focus groups in eight thematic areas. They used this qualitative data to create an assessment of community needs, which they presented during a community visioning session. Next, leaders conducted public planning sessions focused on housing, local entrepreneurship, youth center planning, and community wealth building. Garza noted that the focus on community wealth building was born out of conversations about community safety. In those discussions, residents determined it was not a larger police presence that was needed to increase neighborhood safety, but rather greater community wealth.

The comprehensive quality-of-life plan has the potential to inform the county's planning efforts, Garza described. During the process of creating the plan, the Healthy Richmond team learned that the county was updating its general plan, presenting an opportunity to integrate community plans into the updated general plan, which will drive the development neighborhoods in the county for the next 40 years. Furthermore, 10 acres of neighborhood land will be redeveloped from housing authority property to new use. Garza expressed her hope that the quality-of-life plan would inform the redevelopment of 10 acres of neighborhood land.

Strategies for Power Building in Economic Justice

In the development of the quality-of-life plan,[6] Healthy Richmond used four key drivers of change, Garza said. The first strategy is leveraging the inherent strength of residents. As residents are best equipped to solve their own community needs and problems, Healthy Richmond worked to ensure that it was the residents driving the process. This approach sets the stage for enduring change that is embedded within the community. The next strategy is equipping residents with an understanding of how policy and systems work. In supporting resident leaders, Healthy Richmond provided them with tools and training in effectively navigating the different systems involved in this work. Third, Healthy Richmond attended to bridging cross-cultural connections. The population of the North Richmond community is approximately half Latino and half African American. Garza noted that during the first few meetings, participants divided themselves in the room by race. However, by the end of the project, cross-racial collaboration on presentations was taking place. "It was really amazing to see the work in terms of multiracial, intergenerational backgrounds that can be unified for shared vision for their community," said Garza. This work involved being intentional and sensitive in fostering multiracial alliances and cross-racial solidarity. The fourth strategy is building collective capacity by learning, organizing, and advocating together. The North Richmond residents became a source of strength for one another, incorporating healthy feedback structures to improve the quality of work and connect with each other on a personal level. Garza said that at the end of the project, residents said they felt that they were a family, which she found profoundly meaningful.

Power Building for Health Equity

Healthy Richmond is working for health equity, or "health for all," with an action team supporting power-building strategies for residents. The organization conducted a series of listening sessions with community groups that had difficulty accessing health services across the three health systems in the area: Kaiser Permanente, the county health department,

---

[6] See https://healthyrichmond.net/wp-content/uploads/2020/03QoL-digital-enlish.pfd (accessed July 17, 2021).

and a local community health clinic, examined how these health systems and the culture of the system create barriers. Garza noted that social determinants of health are often the focus in public health; although these are important, the culture of the system is often a problem.

Healthy Richmond created a Health Equity Dine and Learn series by enlisting residents, referred to as "community health advocates," in an ongoing process. These meetings bring community health advocates, health system administrators, and health providers together to discuss approaches, strategies, and best practices in reducing barriers to accessing care. These events are a space in which community health advocates build their power and voice through engaging with the health care leaders making decisions that affect the community. By working to integrate patient voices more fully into the decision-making process, this collaborative effort seeks to change structures in the health care system. This effort has been underway for four years and has poised Healthy Richmond to be actively involved in providing COVID-19 response efforts with the health department. Garza said her organization is pushing the health department to build an infrastructure that can address inequities beyond the COVID-19 pandemic.

Next Steps for Healthy Richmond

Within the context of the nation now reckoning with the historical, generational racism in U.S. systems, Garza stated Healthy Richmond is determining how best to drive its work forward. This involves assessing the current level of collective power and intentionally using strategies to build power across its county. Strategic data and investment in the resident leadership models used in recent years are needed, as well as efforts to develop bridging relationships with systems, system leaders, and champions within systems. Garza noted this piece has been important in the health system in striving for an equitable rollout of the COVID-19 vaccine. She described the last strategy of advancing accountability as the most challenging component of the work. Policy wins in the absence of advancing accountability will not lead to true culture change and reallocation of resources, Garza concluded.

THE POSITIVE DEVIANCE APPROACH

Arvind Singhal, Samuel and Edna Marston Endowed Professor and director of the Social Justice Initiative at The University of Texas at El Paso, discussed the positive deviance approach, which is based on the belief that communities are endowed with the wisdom, the power, and the resources to solve their own problems. He noted that over the past

17 years, he has used this approach to illuminate, address, and solve problems in dozens of communities in dozens of countries, across most continents, including the border area of El Paso, Texas, where he lives. He illustrated the concepts behind this approach with stories of uncommon perspectives given by historical figures, before giving an example of what this approach looks like in practice (Singhal, in press).

Paraphrasing Lao Tzu, a Chinese philosopher from ancient times, Singhal said that in the positive deviance approach, the role of the expert/outsider/interventionist/change agent is to "Go to the people. Live with them. Learn from them. Love them. Start with what they know. Build with what they have." The fundamental premise of the positive deviance approach is that regardless of the issue, and no matter its complexity, there exist people in every community who have already solved the problem. This applies to issues such as food insecurity and malnutrition, low rates of cancer screening, poor diabetes control, teenage pregnancy, high school dropout rates, hospital acquired infections, and other topics (Singhal and Dura, 2009; Singhal et al., 2010). Furthermore, Singhal contended that not only do people exist who have solved the problem, they have done so while facing the highest odds and with no additional resources. The positive deviance approach assumes this is possible through a "flipped" way of thinking that involves asking questions that have not been previously asked, while also asking and acting in a new way. To describe this further, Singhal provided three examples.

Narrative Examples of Positive Deviance Thinking

President Abraham Lincoln is said to have been asked by a soldier: "Mr. President, you are tall. How tall are you?" Singhal said. President Lincoln's reply was something like "Son, like you, I am tall enough that my feet reach the ground." Singhal noted this is not the way we typically think. Height is usually conceptualized in measurements of length. Lincoln's answer implies that wisdom does not lie with the one who is the tallest or with the president and commander-in-chief; rather, wisdom is commonly distributed. This represents a new way of thinking, said Singhal.

Singhal recounted that when he was 17 years old, he began a correspondence with Mother Teresa and he became a collector of her life stories. One such story dates back to 1974, when Mother Teresa arrived in Washington, DC, and was greeted by hundreds of people. Those welcoming her were holding placards asking if she would join them the following day in a march against the Vietnam War. Mother Teresa is said to have declined to march *against* the war, but said she would be the first to lead a march *for* peace. Mother Teresa was indicating that frames are important, said Singhal. That is, she was suggesting asking a different set of questions. Rather than focusing on the problem, on what is not working, on what are the gaps and needs, people can ask instead: What are we for? What are our assets and strengths? What is working?

Lastly, Singhal told a story of Mahatma Gandhi. When traveling by train, Gandhi always rode in third class. He was often asked by his fellow Indians, "Bapu (Father), why do you travel third class? You are the father of the Indian nation." Gandhi's reply: "I travel third class because, as you know, there is no fourth class." Singhal noted this way of thinking and acting is completely outside the norm.

Practical Application of the Positive Deviance Approach

These three stories illustrate a different way of thinking that can be used in understanding how communities hold the power to solve problems, said Singhal. While the concept of "positive deviance" appeared in literature in the 1960s, Jerry and Monique Sternin were the first to operationalize it in the positive deviance approach.[7] In the early 1990s, the Sternins went to Vietnam to address rampant malnutrition (Sternin and Choo, 2000). Rather than asking, "Why are 65 percent of kids under the age of 5 severely malnourished in Vietnam?" they asked, "Are there children from very poor households who are well nourished?" Singhal stated that living in a probabilistic world, this question seems an impossible one, a question to which no regression equation will lead. Yet, working in 4 communities with 3,000 children under the age of 5, the Sternins found approximately two dozen children (less than 1 percent) were well nourished even though they came from very poor families. This demonstrates that the wisdom to solve malnutrition and provide access to food security already existed among this group of families. These families were the statistical deviants in not fitting the norm, and they were positive deviants in having solved the problem (Singhal, 2010). The positive deviance approach is data driven and allows for determining what is working for those who successfully overcome a problem that also affects others in their communities.

After identifying the positive deviance families, the Sternins then explored what these families were doing that other families were not. They discovered that some mothers were using the greens of sweet potato plants and tiny shrimp and crabs from the rice fields, and adding them to the meals. These resources were accessible to all but not part of what children were typically fed. Furthermore, the Sternins learned that some mothers were actively feeding their children to ensure that no food was

---

[7] More information about the evolution of the positive deviance approach is available at https://positivedeviance.org/background (accessed February 24, 2021).

wasted; this behavior was not the norm, as most children were left to eat by themselves. Some mothers were breaking meals into smaller portions, feeding children three to four times per day, rather than twice per day. Smaller meals led to better assimilation of nutrients. Singhal said that while the natural inclination is to tell others about nuggets of wisdom (i.e., best practices) once they are gleaned, the positive deviance approach involves yet another difference from the norm. Instead of telling or showing people new information, the approach involves creating the conditions for people to act out these newly discovered, but uncommon and replicable, behaviors (Singhal and Svenkerud, 2019). In this case, mothers were asked to forage for sweet potato greens and tiny shrimp and crabs, and to bring these to cooking sessions. The mothers attended these sessions and cooked together. They actively fed their children and tracked their children's progress. Within a span of 5 years, 85 percent of those Vietnamese children who were involved in the initiative were well nourished (Pascale et al., 2010). Singhal remarked that these communities in Vietnam solved their problem through their own wisdom and resources. Singhal concluded his remarks with a quote from Robert Frost: "We dance 'round in a ring and suppose, but the secret sits in the middle and knows."

DISCUSSION

Effect of Personal Narrative on Career

Rodríguez opened the discussion with a quote from Spanish philosopher José Ortega y Gasset: "Yo soy yo y mi circunstancia, y si no la salvo a ella no me salvo yo" (Ortega y Gasset, 1914). She translated this as, "I am myself and my circumstance. If I do not articulate it, I cannot explain who I am." With that quote in mind, Rodríguez asked each speaker to share how their circumstance, journey, elders, and community have shaped their work and who they are.

Styles responded that people rarely consider how ancestors' work, trauma, and love for community have shaped the work currently carried out by social justice workers. She provided a brief family history, beginning with her grandfather, who was a police commissioner in Northern California and served as a liaison between the Black Panther Party and his community. Styles's father was a Black Panther, and she speculated that dinner conversations in a household with a police commissioner and a member of the Black Panther Party must have been interesting. Her father became the vice president of the National Association for the Advancement of Colored People, and she grew up under that pulpit. Styles described that "breathing in" that history affirms her work and serves as a reminder to constantly be willing to learn from one's community. She noted that her grandfather was a leader who used his capacity to listen to his community, allowing it to shape the way he moved through the world. For example, he provided economic resources and hired people within his community to work in the stores he built. Styles said she uses his memory as an invitation to continue to do this work in a conscious way that prioritizes listening.

Singhal recounted that while he was a visiting professor at the Rollins School of Public Health at Emory University, the Dalai Lama spoke on campus and began his talk by saying that every time he is on a university campus, he is reminded that the buildings were created to cultivate habits of the head. The Dalai Lama asked, "In addition to these institutions that cultivate habits of the head, where are the institutions, the frameworks, and models that create the conditions for cultivating the habits of the heart?" The longest journey that every person takes, the Dalai Lama continued, a journey which may not even be completed in a lifetime—is the sacred distance between the head and the heart. Referring to the prior examples of Lao Tzu, Abraham Lincoln, Mother Teresa, and Mahatma Gandhi, Singhal said they were all able to connect the head and heart. People working in the space of power building should challenge themselves to create the conditions to connect the head and the heart, Singhal suggested. The conceptualization of power, Singhal believes needs to be reframed as "power to" and "power with" instead of the normative frame of "power over."

Garza recalled that her grandmother immigrated to the United States as an orphaned child, her parents having died of tuberculosis and her siblings separated from one another. She eventually started a family in the town of Tulare in the San Joaquin Valley in California. Garza's parents met in Tulare while working as farm laborers alongside their parents. They moved to Los Angeles, where her father became a commercial artist. However, he encountered many inequities in his field and to challenge them, her father became a union organizer, striving to make Spanish-speaking artists visible. Garza's mother had three children and then dedicated herself to becoming a public health nurse, earning her registered nursing degree when Garza was in high school. Garza said that she grew up watching her parents pay attention to what was happening in their community.

When she applied to the School of Social Welfare at the University of California, Los Angeles, Garza wrote about the trips to a park in downtown Los Angeles with her father and her siblings. They would sit on a park bench and watch the world around them, seeing poverty and homelessness, but also seeing beauty and the joy of immigrants recreating in the park. Garza attributes the fact that she and one of her siblings became social workers to these trips. She recalled being a "feisty child," with an internal fire about injustice burning inside her. In elementary school, one of her teachers called her parents to tell them that Garza became upset every time history and poverty were discussed. Even as a child, she wanted to change economic injustice. During her elementary and junior high school years, busing was still taking place in an attempt to integrate schools and address school inequities. Garza described watching the Democratic primary presidential debate on June 27, 2019, in which candidate Kamala Harris recounted being a child bused to school as part of an integration effort, and reacting, "Yes, me too!" Garza described her childhood experience of seeing the white community fighting—and winning—against integration attempts in the school system. She also witnessed bitter fights among students on campus as children acted on the messages they were getting from their parents. Garza said she cannot separate her soul from social justice and race equity work. Having been pushed out of systems after being labeled a "community advocate," she noted that many colleagues have advised her to separate herself from her work. She has been told, "You are not what you do." To this, she responds, "Well, I actually am, in this case." Garza said she enjoys being on the outside and creating pathways for residents to be in the room where change efforts happen, pushing back on systems that have not made substantial strides in cultural change. "I hope that I can remain humble and serve the residents for the rest of my life," she stated.

Documenting Community History

Rodríguez asked how lessons learned can be passed down and carried forward. She noted her dislike for a quote often attributed to Winston Churchill: "History is written by the victors." The implication of this quote is that history is not always grounded in facts but rather in the winners' interpretation of those facts. She prefers a quote by Nigerian writer Chinua Achebe, who said, "Until the lions have their own historians, the history of the hunt will always glorify the hunter." Rodríguez asked how to ensure that the histories of the communities served are remembered and documented.

Styles explained that the first phase of the CARE model uses a timeline of injustice. When MEASURE works with a community, it spends days or even weeks developing a timeline of how the community has suffered from enslavement of their people, caging of their children, or other injustices that affect the problem the community is seeking to change. This process, which takes place before considering possible solutions, results in a document the team creates with the community and is eventually made into a poster. The intent is to make the history tangible and shareable, facilitating the community and its members ability to communicate their stories.

Garza noted that Healthy Richmond's website includes examples of the case studies and curricula that the organization has created, in addition to a video that residents produced. She said community members need avenues for voicing what they see as important. For example, when residents wanted to present their quality-of-life plan at a planning commission meeting, the county planning department said their attendance was unnecessary and they would ensure all commissioners received a copy. However, Garza knew the community needed to present their plan in person at the meeting, so she pushed for that to happen, and the presentation had a visible impact on the commissioners. She encouraged every unincorporated community to engage in a planning process similar to this. Garza said that organizers can facilitate the creation of spaces for residents to make their own documents, videos, and messaging and help them access avenues to present these materials in counties and cities.

Singhal pointed out that much discourse focuses on evidence-based practice. He believes the notion of "practice-based evidence" needs to be elevated (Singhal and Svenkerud, 2018). Positive deviance is simply a variation in practice that creates the conditions for something unique to a community to be acknowledged, identified, and amplified. A language shift can help root practice in this approach, he added.

5

From Vision to Action: Effective Ways to Support Grassroots Community Power Building

---

CHAPTER HIGHLIGHTS

- While organizing and base building are central for historically excluded populations to have power, agency, and voice, they alone are insufficient to gain influence over decision makers; an ecosystem of capacities is required to build power. (Vaidya)
- Policy is downstream from power. (Han)
- Researchers can best support community power groups by (1) focusing on shared learning, not program evaluation, interventions, or disseminating expertise; (2) centering power, race, and inequality, and recognizing the uncertain, dynamic contexts within which the communities act; and (3) acting toward making the possible more plausible, not just accepting the necessity of the probable. (Han)
- Relationships play an important role in power building, and there is value in investing time to develop them. (Fernandes, James, Vaidya)
- Funders should focus on the organization's strategies, learning needs, and desired outcomes rather than driving their own agenda or falling back on easily measured metrics. (Fernandes, Frey)
- Power building should be approached with a transformational perspective, as opposed to a transactional or siloed approach. (Ho, James)
- When communities have power and self-determination, they can define problems, identify solutions, and carry out systems transformation. (James)

The fourth session of the workshop focused on approaches to power building that place relationships, community voice and self-determination, and the true transfer of power in the center of the discussion. The session had three objectives:

1. Become familiar with the community power-building ecosystem, developed through recent research by the Equity Research Institute of the University of Southern California (USC).
2. Expand the collective understanding of effective principles, research, or tools to advance community power-building efforts led by low-income Black, Indigenous, and people-of-color communities.
3. Learn how leading practitioners are partnering with grassroots communities to advance their long-term agendas for structural change.

Aditi Vaidya, senior program officer at the Robert Wood Johnson Foundation (RWJF), moderated the session.

Vaidya introduced the session as an exploration into how community actions fit into a broader ecosystem of community power in changing the economic, social, and political conditions in neighborhoods. The session was designed to highlight effective principles, research, and tools used to advance community power-building efforts by participants with expertise across a range of domains, including funding, strategy, research, and community organizing.

COMMUNITY POWER-BUILDING ECOSYSTEM

Vaidya noted that the challenges of recent years, including the global COVID-19 pandemic, have been met with a rise of community organizing—particularly among low-income Black, Indigenous, and people-of-color communities. In recent years, successful power-building efforts have initiated changes targeting the root causes of inequities at the local level. In 2020, power building led to a visible amplification of demands for racial and economic justice and for voter participation, particularly among Black, Asian, and Latinx communities. Vaidya said power-building groups have played a critical role in protecting and helping local communities with immediate needs during the pandemic, from fighting evictions to accessing food and shelter.

Vaidya noted a rich body of growing research that supports community power building (Caring Across Generations, 2020; Han, 2020; Human Impact Partners and Right to the City Alliance, 2020; Pastor et al., 2020;

Speer et al., 2020; USC Dornsife Equity Research Institute, 2020). RWJF funded Lead Local, a collaborative effort that spent 2 years producing some of the most up-to-date research on how community power building advances health equity.[1] Manuel Pastor and the team at the USC Equity Research Institute have studied social movements and grassroots community-organizing efforts for more than 20 years, and they were partners in Lead Local. Using this body of research—which includes research led by community power-building groups themselves—RWJF has developed a definition of community power (see Box 5-1).

Power is a multidimensional construct involving an ecosystem of the strategies, processes, and partnerships that are required to build it, said Vaidya. The Equity Research Institute developed a model of this ecosystem. This model is rooted in the understanding that organizing and base building are central for historically excluded populations to have power, agency, and voice, but alone they are insufficient to gain influence over decision makers. Hence, power building requires an ecosystem of capacities. At the center of the model are the concepts of organizing and base building, with other components stemming outward from that center. These include

- advocacy and policy;
- research, both scientific and legal;
- communications, culture shifting, and narrative change;
- alliance and coalitions;
- leadership development; and
- organizational development, infrastructure, and funders.

BOX 5-1
Robert Wood Johnson Foundation's
Definition of Community Power

Community power is the ability of communities most affected by structural inequities to develop, sustain, and grow an organized base of people who act together through democratic structures to set agendas, shift public discourse, influence decision makers, and cultivate ongoing relationships of mutual accountability to change systems and advance health equity.

SOURCE: Vaidya presentation, January 28, 2021.

---

[1] More information about Lead Local, including full reports of findings, is available at https://www.lead-local.org (accessed March 2, 2021).

Quoting Rashad Robinson, president of Color of Change, Vaidya said "The power to define what is needed is the power to shape what is delivered." Organizing for systemic change therefore involves supporting communities to define what they deserve and need, then working with them to build the infrastructure, accountability, narrative change, and organization required to obtain it. Research, resourcing, leadership development, and other functions are critical to supporting, organizing, and base building as part of the community power ecosystem, Vaidya added, and allies in various roles connect to this ecosystem in different ways.

PARTNERSHIPS BETWEEN RESEARCHERS AND COMMUNITY GROUPS

Hahrie Han, professor and director of the Stavros Niarchos Foundation (SNF) Agora Institute and the P3 Research Lab at Johns Hopkins University (JHU), discussed how problems of power require bringing the motivation and authority to make change into alignment. She described the role of research in supporting community power groups and outlined effective approaches to this research. Her guidance was informed by her work directing the SNF Agora Institute, which is dedicated to strengthening global democracy with a particular focus on civil society organizations, and the JHU P3 research lab, which is named for its focus on understanding how to make the participation of ordinary people *possible, powerful,* and *probable*. This research involves finding ways to harness the resources of the academy to help strengthen community organizers' efforts to promote community power building and health equity.

Personal Narrative

Han recounted her family history and its influence on her career in power building. Her parents immigrated to the United States as refugees from North Korea. Growing up in Texas, she watched her parents try to "make it" in the United States, a concept they were trying to define in a foreign land. Wanting to become part of the American culture, they went on family trips to national parks, visiting sights such as Mount Rushmore, because they thought that was what Americans were supposed to do.

Han's parents did not discuss politics, social justice, or social issues. However, she learned from observing her parents that transformation is not only possible, it is a way of life. She saw immigrants and people of all kinds remaking themselves, their families, and the world around them. She discovered politics in college through happenstance engagement with a student organization. When she completed her degree, Han worked in electoral politics, seeing it as a pathway of transformation in society. However, one of the first lessons she learned in electoral politics is that policy is downstream from power. She wanted to work on issues like health equity, education justice, and racial equity that were pivotal in shaping her Texas childhood. However, she learned that in the political system, the issue of power precedes all policy matters. She shifted her focus to doing research that would enable her to learn with a variety of groups about how to exercise power for the outcomes most important to them; this led her to the field of power building.

Alignment for Power

A first step to understanding how to make social change is to clarify an organization's theory of change, Han explained. She remarked that different kinds of social problems require different kinds of solutions. For example, some problems need technological solutions. When polio was a widespread problem, a polio vaccine was needed. Some problems need a shifting framework of incentive—for instance, some people believe that incentivizing people to go to the gym can address problems like obesity. Other problems are problems of information that can be solved when the appropriate alignment of motivation and authority exist. For instance, in the past, doctors advised parents to lay their babies on their stomachs to sleep, believing that practice was healthiest for babies. However, when the doctors' understanding shifted and they realized it is actually healthier for infants to sleep on their backs, they created a campaign to raise awareness of these shifting health guidelines. The Back-to-Sleep campaign was effective in significantly reducing rates of sudden infant death syndrome over time.[2] Han remarked that this campaign was successful because the people who needed to make the change (parents) had both the motivation and the authority to do so. Once provided with information from their doctors about the needed change, parents were highly motivated to do what is best for their children and they had the authority to lay their children on their backs to sleep. Han suggested that problems of power exist when the motivation to make change and the authority to make change are not aligned. This occurs when people who are in great need of change—often frontline communities—do not have the authority to make change. Conversely, when people who have the authority to make

---

[2] The 1994 Back-to-Sleep campaign increased the number of babies sleeping on their backs from 17 percent to 73 percent. Sudden infant death syndrome decreased from a rate of 4,700 U.S. infant deaths in 1993 to 2,063 in 2010. See https://www.aap.org/en-us/advocacy-and-policy/aap-health-initiatives/7-great-achievements/Pages/Reducing-Sudden-Infant-Death-with-Back-to-.aspx (accessed March 10, 2021).

a change are not motivated to do so, the result is a lack of alignment that constitutes a power problem.

Researcher Support of Community Power Groups

Han said that the "stickiest" social problems pertaining to equity are characterized by a misalignment of motivation and authority. These problems of power will not be solved by merely giving people more information, improving technology, or streamlining incentives. Instead, people must act together in coordinated efforts to achieve desired change. Both the P3 lab and the SNF Agora Institute study how to strengthen the processes of people acting together. The P3 lab works with community groups across the United States, including the AMOS Project in Ohio,[3] Living United for Change in Arizona,[4] New Virginia Majority in Virginia,[5] and ISAIAH in Minnesota.[6] Most of these groups act as statewide, independent, political power organizations focused on addressing multiple issues with particular constituencies. They work to elevate the voices of these constituencies and build power in the political system. P3 partners with these groups to sharpen their practice via research efforts, she added.

The role of a P3 researcher extends beyond evaluating an organization's program, said Han. As researchers, they seek to tackle questions at the forefront of the organization's strategic dilemmas and the minds of organizers. They also co-create learning systems with the organization, sharpening the organizers' practice and informing an understanding of how community power relates to issues such as health equity. Additionally, the researchers try to make the organizers' work visible in ways that enable learning not only for the organization but for the broader community. For example, researchers may map the organization's power networks or examine the ways in which the organization has been building its constituency over time. These visualizations of the organizing help organizers to do three things: (1) identify where they have successfully built constituency and where they have not, (2) determine their place within the power networks in which they work, and (3) define the role these community power groups play in the larger ecosystem that was presented by Vaidya. Moreover, P3 strives to push the boundaries of strategic

---

[3] More information about the AMOS Project is available at https://theamosproject.org (accessed March 19, 2021).

[4] More information about Living United for Change is available at https://luchaaz.org (accessed March 19, 2021).

[5] More information about the New Virginia Majority is available at https://www.newvirginiamajority.org (accessed March 19, 2021).

[6] More information about ISAIAH in Minnesota is available at https://isaiahmn.org (accessed March 19, 2021).

thinking, both among the community power groups themselves as well as among scholars. Han said that over time, P3 identified a characteristic that most differentiates the most effective community power groups from others: constantly operating in learning mode. Thus, she contended that researchers have an important role to play in cultivating, developing, and supporting learning within and among community partners.

Lessons Learned: Building Partnerships Between Researchers and Community Power Groups

Han remarked that being good allies to community power groups is challenging because it requires iteration over time to learn the best approaches. In building partnerships between researchers and community power groups, P3 has identified three lessons about how to provide support effectively. The first lesson is to focus on shared learning. When considering how research is approached, the researcher is often viewed as controlling the intellectual directions of the relationship. For instance, the researchers set up a research design, and may randomize subjects into treatment and control arms. A variety of researcher-controlled arenas can exist, which is complicated for organizations that are working in dynamic power environments in the field, she noted. Han and her team are intentional about simultaneously seeking to meet the highest standards of academic rigor to develop knowledge and learning, but also co-creating and sharing control across the entire partnership. Thus, groups working on the issue of power and the scholarly research community are both learning through a bidirectional flow of expertise. This understanding is fundamental to creating effective partnerships between researchers and community power groups, she added.

The second lesson is to place questions of power, race, and inequality in the center of the discussion. Han remarked that over the years, she has worked with a number of different groups that are each unique in their own ways. However, the commonality among them is that no matter what issue they are working on, which constituency, or what kind of a political arena, they are all operating within an uncertain, dynamic context. That uncertainty provides an important frame for the research. It is not by coincidence that these groups have historically struggled to build power within the political system, she said. This underscores the need to focus, from the outset, on questions about why systems have been structured to disadvantage certain groups, and how these groups are constantly navigating uncertain contexts. To support the work these community power groups are doing, the focus should be placed on issues related to power, race, and inequality; otherwise, it is easy for projects to move in tactical directions that are not necessarily fruitful.

Han described the third lesson using a quote from a twelfth-century Jewish theologian, Maimonides: "Hope is the belief in the plausibility of the possible, not the necessity of the probable." If one looks only at the data on social change and the role of community power, the overwhelming response to any change effort in American politics is stasis, she said. The status quo is the most likely outcome whenever people, no matter who they are, try to make change. Effectively supporting community power groups to initiate change requires a shift from thinking about what is probable to envisioning what is possible, she said. Researchers can help groups imagine a different kind of future and then work to make that future a reality. Han added that the role of research and learning is to cultivate and sustain that imagination, as well as to substantiate it through learning partnerships.

CURRENT POWER-BUILDING STRATEGIES AND APPROACHES

Vaidya commented that the lessons highlighted by Han fit into the community power-building ecosystem model. As LaTosha Brown, co-founder of the Black Voters Matter Fund, and Ai-jen Poo, co-founder and executive director at the National Domestic Workers Alliance, detailed in their presentations at the start of the workshop, this work is grounded in human value and addressing the erosion of human value. Practical research and technology have functions within the ecosystem, as do engaging local partners in shared learning and forming relationships across areas of expertise and varying roles, Vaidya maintained. Noting the variety of professional backgrounds present, she invited each of the remaining speakers to describe their sector or field and reflect on any ideas shared by Han that resonated with their own experiences.

Power Building at the State Level

Ethan Frey, program officer at the Ford Foundation, began his career as a political and labor organizer focused on workplace and electoral campaigns.[7] He is currently part of the Ford Foundation's Cities and States team, leading a grantmaking initiative. The program's focus is supporting multiracial coalitions that are led by people of color and seeking to build statewide governing power. From states' rights to President Reagan's devolution revolution, U.S. states hold increasing political and economic

---

[7] More information about the Ford Foundation is available at https://www.fordfoundation.org (accessed February 28, 2021).

power over communities that is often out of reach for grassroots community organizers.[8] States exert control over a range of issues including the minimum wage, Medicaid expansion, and various rights and protections for vulnerable communities. Therefore, in order for communities to have real power, they must attain power at the state level, Frey said. His team examines how grassroots organizations can most effectively build power at the state level.

Referencing Han's point that policy is downstream from power, Frey commented that unless policy changes address underlying power dynamics, policy will eventually revert to its original condition. Thus, to create conditions for durable, lasting change at the state level, his organization's strategy is to rearrange and reorganize state power dynamics. Working in New York, Michigan, Minnesota, Texas, Louisiana, and Florida, it supports multiracial coalitions. These coalitions are accountable to organized constituency groups that have the ability to align other forces and capacities in their ecosystems around a shared strategy. Efforts to operationalize strategy through learning and building new infrastructure are under way in several of these coalitions.

Given his team's focus on effecting change at the state level by partnering with grassroots organizations, Frey emphasized the importance of clarity around strategy and desired power shifts. For instance, efforts to build power via the narrative arena and by shaping policy through state legislatures require clarity about desired power shifts in those domains. Building the capacity within an organization to measure and learn from the changes initiated in those domains is challenging, however. Frey continued that funders and political donors often put pressure on organizations to measure easily quantifiable metrics such as numbers of contacts or activities, but these metrics are often disconnected from community organization strategies. He emphasized that funders should focus instead on evaluating an organization's strategies, identifying the power they want to build, and being a good partner in that work.

Seizing the Transformative Moment

Mimi Ho, executive director at the Movement Strategy Center (MSC), has been a community and labor organizer for 20 years. She stated that the current historical moment warrants the abandonment of a siloed approach and a significant transformation of "business as usual." To effectively address inequities and community disparities, people should

---

[8] The devolution revolution was a movement started by Ronald Reagan in the 1980s that involved the gradual return of power from the federal level to the states.

collaborate across fields.[9] She noted that the knowledge and policy proposals needed for this transformation are in place: it is only power that is missing. Power must be transformed in concrete ways at the national level, in state houses, and in local jurisdictions, said Ho. Furthermore, to truly accelerate change and power in the present moment, a transformation of human values and human spirit is needed. This unique moment presents great opportunity to leverage both the disruption caused by the worldwide crisis of the COVID-19 pandemic and the beauty of the human spirit that has surfaced in response. Capturing the cultural and transformative moment—and combining it with rigorous power-building strategies—can lead to true change. However, Ho posited that change at a magnitude that affects large segments of the population will only be achieved by combining the rigor of power building with connection to the dynamic human spirit.

Ho remarked that the wide variety of speakers at the workshop reflects a shift away from the silos that traditionally characterize this work. For example, community organizers are experimenting with narrative change and cultural change, while policy experts and researchers are leveraging their power in service to community. Furthermore, community organizing is shifting to true community power building. She said that community organizations need to center people within communities at a much larger scale. Pushing the boundaries of ambition would help to achieve the type and scale of power that is sufficient to accelerate change. She added that this change cannot be incremental—exponential change is essential right now.

The Role of Self-Determination and Ideology in Power Building

Julie Fernandes, associate director for institutional accountability and individual liberty at the Rockefeller Family Fund (RFF), spent most of her career as an advocate before becoming a funder.[10] She described herself as a civil rights lawyer who loves research for learning and who engages in a continual effort to improve her practice to better serve everyone. For years, she worked as a civil rights lobbyist in Washington, DC, supporting bills focused on people of color, women, LGBTQ (lesbian, gay, bisexual, transexual, queer), and other groups. Some of these efforts were

---

[9] Significant recent events at the time of the workshop included the COVID-19 pandemic, the Black Lives Matter movement for racial justice and equality, the historic turnout for the recent 2020 presidential election, and the storming of the U.S. Capitol that took place on January 6, 2021.

[10] More information about the Rockefeller Family Fund is available at https://www.rffund.org (accessed March 1, 2021).

successful, but others were not. In one case, while working on a big campaign, she felt confident that their efforts would be successful because her group believed that they had the answer to the issue at hand and the necessary allies in place. Still, the measure they were working on failed. While debriefing, she and her group identified a lack of power as underpinning that loss. In spite of having elite access in Washington, DC, her group was disconnected from the communities on whose behalf they purported to operate. Fernandes said without truly knowing what the communities needed, her group was not authentically connected to the work. This issue of disconnection made her realize she needed to dedicate time to understanding where real power lies. She asked herself whether communities have power, and if not, why not? If so, why was the power not resulting in change?

To answer these questions, Fernandes traveled around the United States, talking to groups in different states about what they did not like in the failed bill. If they did like the bill, they were asked about barriers that kept them from helping to ensure it passed. She gained valuable insights through this process, including the realization that policy is downstream from power. Her background in voting, democracy, and elections work has led to her belief that outcomes are determined by self-determination and communities. She noted that in conversations with progressives about democracy and power building in communities, she is often met with resistance. Some progressives express worry that their agenda may not pass using a community-led approach. However, the goal of passing an agenda developed without community input lacks the values of self-determination and community power. In contrast, an approach rooted in self-determination and democracy views the communities of color affected by the problem as those most intimately familiar with it; therefore, these communities would likely have the more effective ideas about how to solve it. Fernandes said her role is supporting communities with the tools needed to carry out solutions. Entities dedicated to constituent power building may need support in developing strategies to move that power toward achieving desired outcomes, she added.

Fernandes noted that narrative is a focus of her work with the Democracy and Power Innovation Fund at RFF. A major area of inquiry is understanding how people of color—African Americans, other Black Americans, Latinos, Asian Americans, and other groups—think about themselves and their power. This understanding can contribute to supporting people in recognizing their full power and helping them use it to make change happen via collective action. Fernandes said that when she talks to people in the Black community, she often hears questions such as: How am I going to change anything? What am I going to do when the whole system is not built for me? She suggested that people's thoughts can make them feel either powerful or not powerful. People can be more effectively supported to feel powerful enough to lean in, act collectively, and make change happen if efforts are made from the outset to understand their thoughts, including people's political ideologies, beliefs, and assumptions that determine how they behave politically—not merely in terms of voting, but also in terms of civic engagement—to make change happen. Fernandes stated that in the work around democracy and elections, there is very little research about nonwhite people, yet many assumptions are made about how people who are not white think and operate. She and her team are working to break down these assumptions to arrive at true understanding, then use that knowledge to support organizing, power building, civic engagement, and the role of narrative throughout those processes.

Lastly, Fernandes highlighted the cultural aspect of organizing, which includes both narrative and ideology. Narrative comes into play both in terms of understanding the narratives people hold and in creating powerful narratives that operate to make change happen. Ideological assumptions are constructed over time and driven by culture. People adopt these constructed ideologies without even knowing it, she said. Power building involves deconstructing ideologies that strengthen the status quo, while also creating new ideologies that speak to people and bring them to a more progressive place. Speaking to the strength of ideology, Fernandes gave the example of the shift in understanding of the second amendment of the U.S. Constitution. She said that when she became a lawyer in the 1990s, most people did not interpret the second amendment as giving everyone the right to own any type of gun. The majority of people did not believe that protected gun ownership rights extended to assault weapons. However, for many people, that ideology has shifted to a belief that the second amendment does provide for the right to own assault weapons. Another example is the ideology that chief executive officers are entitled to the profits of their companies. Although all employees contribute to a company's success, the default American ideology tends to be that "capitalists earn the money and workers just get the scraps," said Fernandes. That sentiment is ideology, not truth, just as anti-Black racism is an ideology. Power building involves understanding how to shift ideology around who has value, what matters, what capital means, and how it influences the world, she maintained.

Fernandes asserted that the role of ideology and culture is well understood by the political right. She referenced seminars in which conservatives emphasize "winning on culture" because culture is ideology, and culture and ideology are, in turn, policy. She urged progressives to embrace the transformative potential of culture and ideology, because they are forces greater than individual policy wins.

Transformation and Forms of Power

Taj James, co-founder of Full Spectrum Capital Partners and co-founder, former executive director, and current board member of the Movement Strategy Center, described this discussion as reminiscent of Martin Luther King, Jr.'s assertion that there will be no equity and no justice without a revolution in values.[11] King said, "When machines and computers, profit motives, and property rights are considered more important than people, the giant triplets of racism, extreme materialism, and militarism are incapable of being conquered" (King, 1967). James remarked that the challenges we face are essentially spiritual and cultural challenges pertaining to fundamental questions of what it means to be human: What is the value of life? What is the nature of our relationships with each other? What is our place in the cosmos? He noted that activists Grace Lee Boggs, Michelle Alexander, and Reverend William Barber have revisited King's tradition of centralizing the role of culture and values in deepening a broader transformation.

Describing himself as "a community organizer in recovery," James served as co-director at MSC for many years, which was a role he shared with Ho. The focus of that work was to learn how to approach power building with a transformational perspective, as opposed to a transactional or siloed approach. The California Endowment collaborated with MSC to design and launch Building Healthy Communities, a 10-year initiative focused on health equity. He said that this decade-long process led to his realization that health equity is not simply an issue of public health or education reform; instead, power is the fundamental issue. When communities have power and self-determination, they can define problems, identify solutions, and carry out systems transformation. However, many different definitions of power exist, so developing a precise and rooted understanding of power building is important, he added.

James presented a model of domains of power that pertain to health equity: cultural power, political power, economic power, and, at the intersection of those three domains, integrated and transformative power (see Figure 5-1). Cultural power is the ability to define reality, political power is the ability to define the rules, and economic power is the ability to define relationships. In the philanthropy and social change sphere, emphasis is often placed on political power and, at times, cultural and narrative power are a secondary focus in working to change who the decision makers are. Although real economic power building is foundational, it receives little attention within the nonprofit, philanthropic

---

[11] More information about Full Spectrum Capital Partners is available at https://fullspectrumcapitalpartners.us (accessed March 1, 2021).

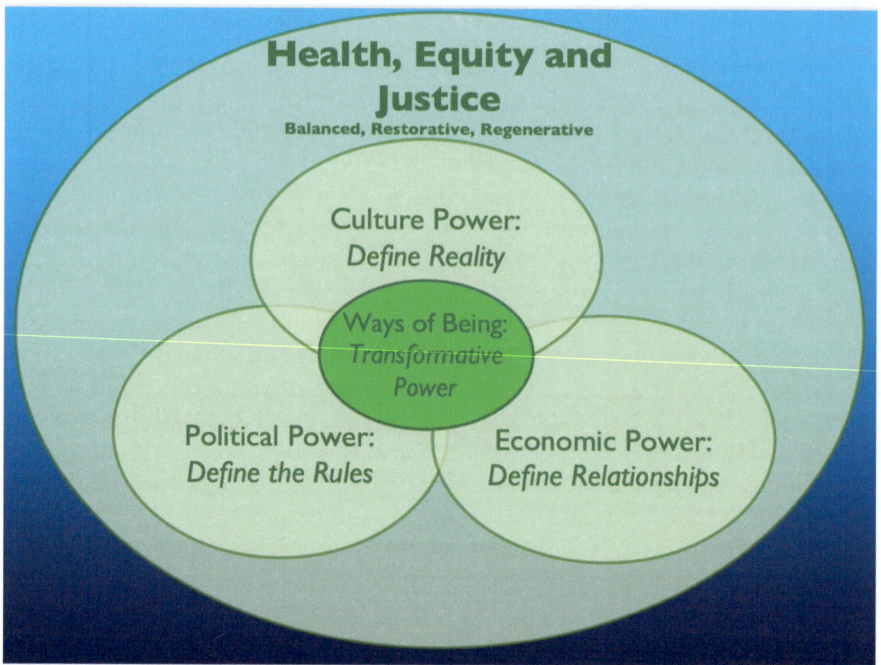

FIGURE 5-1 Domains of power in health, equity, and justice.
SOURCE: James presentation, January 28, 2021.

infrastructure—this is problematic, because political power is reflective of economic power. Many wealthy individuals consider assets to be more important than equity, he noted. Given the power that assets entail, his work focuses what is owned, how it is owned, and who owns it. Power-building strategies should include an economic dimension while strengthening political and cultural power, he continued. While economic power is foundational, cultural power is primary and encompassing. Emphasizing Fernandes's statements about narrative, ideology, and culture, James remarked that the political right has been effective in systematically focusing on narrative and cultural power, because those who define reality are more likely to be able to make rules and change policy. The community power-building ecosystem model presented by Vaidya also pertains to political power, he added. Other frameworks and approaches have also been developed that capture the complexities of cultural power building, economic power building, and integrated or transformative power (see Figure 5-2). He is currently working to use the strength and capacity built around political power as an anchor to integrate with cultural and economic power.

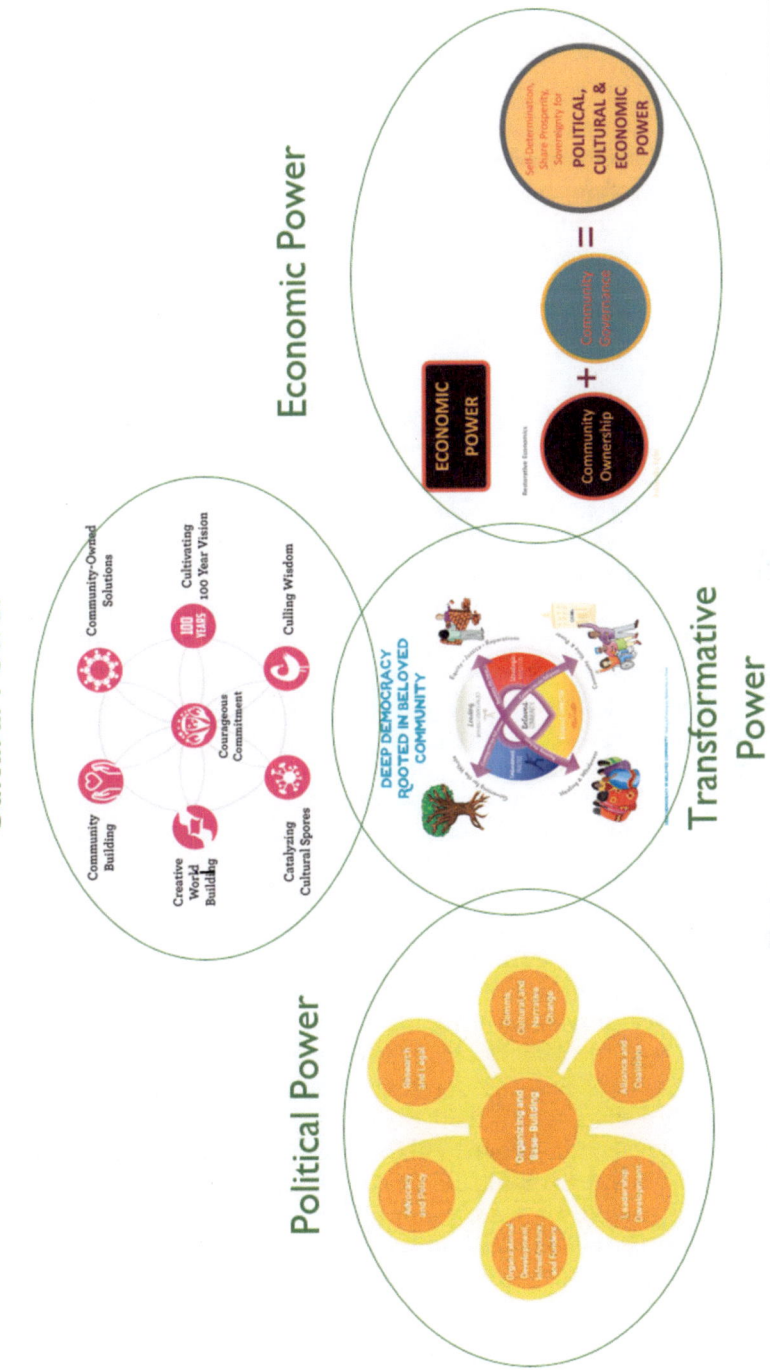

FIGURE 5-2 Approaches to cultural, political, economic, and transformative power building.
SOURCE: James presentation, January 28, 2021.

DISCUSSION

Vaidya commented on the wide variety of approaches to power building that are used in terms of frameworks, definitions, ways that people work together, and the relationships that are built. However, the values of self-determination and centering efforts on organizing and base building appear to be common throughout. The work is grounded in practical implications, determining what is working, what is not working, and the "hard stuff in between," she noted.

Shared Learning Processes

A variety of professionals are working to drive community-held visions forward with action, said Vaidya. Although many multisector collaborations exist between researchers and the grassroots organizing sector, they are not always centered around organizing. Furthermore, the various collaborations do not necessarily work in concert with one another. She asked for practical ways that professionals can approach working together and building relationships with grassroots organizations.

Han provided an example from her collaboration with Faith in Action (formerly known as the People Improving Communities through Organizing or PICO national network), a national network of faith-based, community-organizing groups. Before becoming Faith in Action's national campaigns director, Joy Cushman worked at the New Organizing Institute, an organization that supported community power building across the United States. While at the New Organizing Institute, Cushman invited Han to serve as an evaluator for a grant. They conducted a study, found results that showed the effect of the organization's program, and learned about how to build partnerships. However, both she and Cushman left the partnership feeling their collaboration could have led to deeper learning if not confined by funder-imposed structuring. When Cushman transitioned to Faith in Action, Han and Paul Speer, professor and chair of the Department of Human and Organizational Development at Vanderbilt University, agreed to co-chair a Faith in Action research council that would partner with organizers and federation leaders to create a shared learning agenda through discussions held over the following year. Creating this shared learning agenda began with aligning values, which was a time-intensive process of trust building throughout the team. Next, they identified questions organizers were grappling with that scholars also wanted to understand. These common areas—where learning could be advanced in both fields—became the agenda.

For Han, a turning point was the realization that studying the work of Faith in Action necessitated moving beyond tactical studies toward studies that helped understand if and how Faith in Action was challenging fundamental assumptions about the way the political establishment should be structured. Some of these assumptions, for instance, got at the ways in which narrative power and cultural power were exercised in this work, she added. For example, if it is assumed that communities of color and low-income people cannot be organized or turned out to vote, the entire electoral system is set up in a way that leaves them out. Instead of designing studies that would help people learn about ways to incrementally optimize voter turnout, she and her colleagues developed studies seeking to challenge the fundamental assumptions about the voting behavior of low-income people and communities of color. Thus, the research focused on the fundamental assumptions that structure power in our society, and questions were constructed accordingly. Once these questions were in place, the group then determined how to set up the research to answer them. Han added that the process involved a combination of building buy-in and developing the ability to articulate the assumptions they wanted to challenge or query via research.

The Role of Funding in Power Building

Vaidya asked the funders on the panel how they came to be in their current roles. Furthermore, given the wealth and variety of ideas, she asked how the funders sift through proposals for seeding research, forging new power-building collaborations, and developing power-building plans to develop strategies that align with the focus of their respective foundations.

Fernandes worked in the U.S. Department of Justice under the Obama administration on voting rights and election issues and at the Open Society Foundation as an advisor to grantees on devising advocacy strategy. Realizing the power in money and structuring grantmaking, she began examining how grantmaking can support power-building organizing. She remarked, "How you do grantmaking is as important as whether you do it." Fernandes highlighted the common disconnection between funder-driven work and the questions that are important to organizers. Although it can provide funders with a greater degree of control—which some funders wish to have—it also undermines the ability to advance this work in a meaningful way. Instead, she suggested that these efforts ought to be built around open dialogue about what grantees want and need. However, this level of openness can depend upon establishing a strong relationship, because fear of losing access to funds can discourage grantees from being open about their needs. Fernandes described relationships as the core of effective grantmaking. The grant maker should form relationships with base-building organizations, which involves phone conversations, video meetings, attending meetings the organizers attend, and listening to understand what the organizations need and how they operate. Funders should also form relationships with people who have a thorough understanding of the field and draw from their expertise. Fernandes added that funders should be genuine in this process of relationship building and approach this work as a process of co-creation.

When the Democracy and Power Innovation fund was set up, the founders were intentional about beginning the work with groups they had previously established relationships with, said Fernandes. The fund has the flexibility to open to additional groups. In such cases, they prioritize discovering the group's learning needs and focus on those needs, rather than the funders' interests. The fund then connects groups with researchers to explore those areas. Fernandes emphasized this can be a difficult process, because organizers and funders are drivers who are more accustomed to directing than to co-creating. She reflected, "I am a lobbyist. I am a total driver…but you have to check yourself and walk with humility." Fernandes said she is inspired when working with the groups she collaborates with, because "They know what they want. They know what the problem is, and they know they are in a system where they are devalued."

Frey noted that using private capital to build public power can give rise to dilemmas. For instance, nonprofits are not inherently democratic. Leaders make internal design choices about structuring people and resources that shape power outcomes in the real world. This dynamic is instructive for grant makers in selecting projects while wading through the huge nonprofit industrial complex. Frey remarked that funders trade using their primary resource, private capital. In making selection decisions, he talks with organizations about who their leaders are, how they practice accountability to their leaders, and how this is reflected in the data they are tracking and the learning they are doing. He considers whether people are truly the primary source of the organization's power, which is not a foregone conclusion. It is also helpful to distinguish scale from impact. For example, an organization may have large volumes of outputs and activities that are not translating to improvements. "You can do a lot more with five committed leaders than you can with a million contacts, as a lot of social movements have shown," said Frey.

Cross-Sector Relationship Building

Vaidya highlighted several principles that emerged in the discussion. One is prioritizing shared learning over outcomes-driven, policy-driven conclusions. Another is the role of relationships in power and the value of spending time to build relationships. Despite using various frameworks and different definitions, the panelists commonly discussed grounding their work in everyday people and organizing the base as core elements to power building. From that center, the work is then to determine the best ways to engage with organizing and base building. Vaidya asked the speakers to offer advice to people who are new to organizing and power building about how to build relationships with a sector and engage in shared learning.

James suggested adopting a holistic perspective in thinking about power and communities. One of the greatest barriers between communities and philanthropy is the disparity between the whole, integrated nature of life in community and the segmented, siloed nature of philanthropic institutions, he said. It is possible to avoid the resulting disconnection—which can harm the relationship even when philanthropic organizations have the best of intentions—by identifying a specific, shared focus between the institution and the community (e.g., adolescent health) and to collaborate in a holistic way. James added that philanthropy should increase its emphasis on economic power, treating a grant not as reparations but as a transfer of assets that puts the power of philanthropy into the hands of the community. A different set of health outcomes requires a power transfer; without a transfer of economic power within communities, for example, grants will not accomplish desired outcomes.

Ho stated that this moment requires institutions to leave their silos. Given the collapse of a variety of systems—climate, economic, health, and government—the time is ripe for innovation and building new systems, she said.[12] This can be achieved by building one-on-one relationships and convening across professional fields to center communities in the redesigning of these systems. Furthermore, experts should leverage their assets and positional power to create laboratories that cross sectors and serve a variety of stakeholders. She posited that the next four years will offer a window of opportunity for redesigning systems, with participants in this workshop being uniquely positioned to carry out the necessary change efforts.

Vaidya asked the remaining speakers to share a word or phrase regarding how to approach partnering in grassroots power building. Fernandes highlighted "humility," Frey responded with "relationships," and Han suggested entering into relationships with authenticity.

---

[12] Multiple extreme weather events took place in the United States in 2020, which experts have associated with climate change. The U.S. economy shifted in response to the business shutdowns caused by the COVID-19 pandemic. At the time of the workshop, the United States had the highest numbers of COVID-19 deaths and infections of any country worldwide. See https://coronavirus.jhu.edu/map.html (accessed March 3, 2021). On January 6, 2021, rioters attempted to overturn the 2020 U.S. presidential election by storming the U.S. Capitol to prevent the confirmation of the electoral vote count.

6

Community-Led Transformational Narratives

> **CHAPTER HIGHLIGHTS**
>
> - A community's culture, memories, experiences, and connections form a rich foundation on which to build community-driven efforts. (Ferdinand)
> - Changes in individual behaviors will not undo the health inequities inherent in discrepancies in life expectancy and health outcomes based on zip code. To address root causes, these discrepancies must be traced back to the discriminatory policies, and power dynamics and systems of oppression around race and class must be discussed explicitly. (Llanes Pulido, Petit)
> - Communities are best able to identify barriers and generate solutions; thus, interventions co-created with community members are most effective. (Carrillo, Llanes Pulido, Petit)
> - Institutions and state-level departments can leverage their power to bolster community power building by directing resources to community-driven processes. (Carrillo, Llanes Pulido, Sostaita)
> - Traditional community engagement can be transactional when focused on quantitative metrics regarding event attendance and survey completion. To become transformative, community engagement should center discussions of power and the voices of community members. (Carrillo)

During the fifth session of the workshop, participants highlighted place-based initiatives in creating health equity, discussed effective methods of leveraging power at the community and state levels, and explored the interplay of personal narrative and community power building. Gary Gunderson, vice president for faith and health at Wake Forest Baptist Medical Center, and Arvind Singhal, endowed professor and director of the Social Justice Initiative at The University of Texas at El Paso (UTEP), co-moderated the session.

AGENCY AND COMMUNITY POWER

Gunderson introduced the panelists as agents of community power who navigate power relationships in community settings that are marked by dramatic inequity along predictable lines of race, ethnicity, language, and legal status. He referred to his religious tradition's use of the Greek term *dunamis* to describe the demonstrations of community power evident in the programs led by the panelists. Framing the process of community building as power has not been entirely welcome, even within the National Academies, said Gunderson. Community building is often simplified to a process of creating venues for programs offering best practices, as defined by academic evaluation. This conception overlooks the multi-relevant phenomenon that is power.

The Leading Causes of Life framework centers the agency of every individual in its conceptualization of community (Gunderson and Pray, 2009).[1] The universality of this energy, which some call "spirit," is responsible for the development of morals and individual accountability for choices, said Gunderson. Individual humans, neighborhoods, institutions, and political bodies all have agency. He remarked that this session's speakers facilitate, nurture, provoke, evoke, and align that universal energy—which cannot be introduced to a community; rather, it must be summoned from within the community. At times, this process can be described as "getting institutions of privilege to remove the knee off the neck of community," he said.

Gunderson offered an example from a webinar he had recently participated in, which brought together representatives from public health, a major community coalition, and a health care system in Saint Paul, Minnesota, to discuss how a group of 60 community organizations—most of them faith based—could support the COVID-19 vaccination effort. Curious, he asked the organizer how far her office was from the site of George

---

[1] This assets-based framework focuses away from deficits and causes of death, instead identifying strengths in the following areas: agency, coherence, connection, intergenerativity, and hope.

Floyd's murder.[2] He learned that her office was 10 blocks away from the killing and her clinic was burned during the riots. All 60 organizations were deeply involved in the community's power dynamics, and joining in the community rage and resistance gave them credibility in advancing effective vaccination efforts, Gunderson posited. In spite of this power dynamic's relevance to a major public health effort, the webinar did not discuss it. This session of the present workshop was designed for agents of community power to transparently describe their labor and the art of manifesting community power. Gunderson noted that these stories are not entirely safe to tell nor entirely safe to hear.

Singhal said El Paso, Texas, the border town where he lives, is a magical, bilingual, bicultural, binational environment. Of the 25,000 students attending UTEP, 70 percent are first-generation college students and about 10 percent live across the border in Mexico. The university is near the Walmart where 22 people were killed and 26 were wounded during a shooting on August 3, 2019. El Paso once again made national news in November 2020, when one of the worst COVID-19 surges in the United States required the use of refrigerated morgue trucks. Singhal said health inequities and the number of multigeneration homes contributed to the community's virus surge. Nonetheless, El Paso met the pandemic with action. He recounted recently receiving his COVID-19 vaccination on campus in a campaign organized by the UTEP Schools of Pharmacy and Nursing. The person who administered his vaccination—while mentoring an apprentice in the process—described living across the border and having to leave home at 6:30 a.m. to arrive at work on time. This agency in action is the power and spirit of community, said Singhal, and it is often not mentioned in the national news. He noted that each of the panelists were requested to present an image that represents their efforts to bring forth that energy in their communities.

THE POWER IN HONORING CULTURE

Rashida Ferdinand, founder and executive director at the Sankofa Community Development Corporation, is from the lower Ninth Ward area of New Orleans, Louisiana.[3] In 2008, she started her organization with the goal of improving the quality of life for people in her neighborhood by addressing systemic barriers that cause health inequities and dis-

---

[2] George Floyd was killed on May 25, 2020, by a Minneapolis police officer who pressed his knee on Floyd's neck for nearly 9 minutes. Video footage of his death led to worldwide protests for racial justice and an end to police brutality. In Minneapolis-Saint Paul, protests escalated to riots that involved arson and looting.

[3] More information about Sankofa Community Development Corporation is available at https://sankofanola.org (accessed March 6, 2021).

parities. The organization's mission is to build healthier communities for generations to come. She presented the image of her organization's logo, which features a drawing of the mythical Sankofa bird turning toward its tail feathers. The organization adopted the concept of the Sankofa bird from the Akan people in the Ghana and Sierra Leone areas of West Africa. This mythical creature is said to look over its tail while walking forward, symbolizing the process of looking at the past while finding a future path. The name *Sankofa* was generated from multiple words that have been joined together vernacularly, and it means "go back and fetch."

The Sankofa concept is relevant because people bring culture, history, and knowledge they want to pass on into efforts to move the community forward, said Ferdinand. The people, memories, experiences, and connections within a community form a rich foundation that her group strives to acknowledge and appreciate. While projects, metrics, outcomes, systems, logistics, financials, and all the details of running an organization are at play, the core intention of the work is to focus on people and the quality of their lives, which involves inclusively honoring and respecting where people come from. Ferdinand stated that honoring ancestral culture is a universal concept, and the Sankofa bird—which she has been drawing since she was a child—is one way to symbolize it.

Singhal responded by highlighting a quote he attributed to Nelson Mandela about never forgetting where one comes from and never forgetting about where one is headed: "We owe it to our ancestors" and "we owe it to our children." He noted Ferdinand's acknowledgment of where she came from, where her community is, and the desired generational outcomes for the future.

GO AUSTIN/VAMOS AUSTIN COMMUNITY INITIATIVES

Carmen Llanes Pulido, executive director at Go Austin/Vamos Austin (GAVA), presented a collage of photos from the last large gathering of its coalition in Austin, Texas, before social restrictions related to the COVID-19 pandemic were put into place.[4] The collage included images from a variety of settings, including classrooms, homes, and neighborhoods. One photo captured a walking tour given by community members to institution representatives that highlighted infrastructural challenges faced in the neighborhood. This tour is part of GAVA's community climate resilience work. Other pictures captured house meetings and school events at which participants collaborated on place-based efforts to build community power for health equity. Solutions are designed for the locations

---

[4] More information about Go Austin/Vamos Austin is available at https://www.goaustinvamosaustin.org (accessed March 6, 2021).

where people live, work, learn, play, and worship with the goal of making healthy living accessible and equitable in relevant ways.

Despite much work being performed remotely during the COVID-19 pandemic, GAVA has had a busy and productive year responding to community needs such as access to healthy food and safe physical activity, said Llanes Pulido. The COVID-19 pandemic has disproportionately affected many of the neighborhoods that community organizers are working in, making this work all the more relevant. Llanes Pulido noted the significance of the National Academies of Sciences, Engineering, and Medicine hosting a workshop focused on power, which she viewed as a reflection of the progress achieved through a tremendous amount of action toward community building.

Singhal shared a filmmaker's comment that "The camera denies the existence of what it does not see." If the camera animates and explicates the photographer's focus, he added, GAVA's collage emphasized the importance of conversation and the power of engagement. Gunderson commented that no one in the collage is looking at the camera, instead looking at each other in earnest dialogue. Singhal replied that this reflects "ubuntu," the African philosophy of "I am because we are"—that one's sense of self is shaped by relationships.

CHURCH-BASED COMMUNITY SERVICES

Daniel Sostaita, pastor at Iglesia Cristiana Sin Fronteras (ICSF), spoke about the work his ministry carries out in Winston-Salem, North Carolina.[5] He commented that while people may view Jesus as someone with all the answers, he was actually a man who asked many questions. Notably, Jesus approached others with the question, "What can I do for you?" Striving to follow Jesus's example, Sostaita said he centers his practice around that question.

ICSF is part of a coalition that provides a number of services to the community. In collaboration with Wake Forest Baptist Health (WFBH), mobile health clinic services—including COVID-19 testing—are available at the church on a weekly basis. Through a partnership with two local hospitals, WFBH and Novant Health, a mammogram program is offered at the church twice per year to women who lack health insurance because of their undocumented status. Additionally, the church hosts events offering free flu shots, hot meals, a clothing closet, and, during the COVID-19 pandemic—free face masks. In collaboration with Love Out Loud, Second Harvest Food Bank, and other partners, ICFS provides grab-and-go meals.

---

[5] More information about Iglesia Cristiana Sin Fronteras (Christian Church Without Borders) is available at https://www.iglesiacristianasinfronteras.org (accessed March 4, 2021).

Furthermore, the church is part of a task force composed of organizations such as FaithHealth, the Forsyth County Department of Public Health, Red Latina (CBF NC), and Radio Onda de Amor (Wave of Love). The task force provides outreach services in which food, face masks, and health information are offered in various neighborhoods. A weekly program on Radio Onda de Amor provides radio listeners with conversation and resources around health. ICFS partners with the Winston-Salem Foundation and the Jefferson Christian Church to provide financial assistance to undocumented immigrants for needs such as food, rent, and utilities. The church also links specific populations, such as women who have experienced domestic violence and boys who have substance abuse needs, to therapy services. Sostaita said he centers Jesus's question of "What can I do for you?" in organizing this range of support.

Gunderson described Sostaita's work as releasing the power of the community to counter oppression. He offered an example of Sostaita organizing 250 community members to hold the school system accountable in regard to the radical disparities seen during the COVID-19 pandemic. Therefore, Sostaita goes beyond organizing services for the community in amplifying the community voice to hold local politicians accountable for educational administrative decisions. Gunderson said the art of encouraging the flow of community power is versatile, sometimes involving partnering to provide mobile health services at the church and other times influencing the school system to hire more bilingual staff. All of these actions are expressions of agency and of power.

POLICY ADVOCACY FOR HEALTH EQUITY

Christine Petit is an active leader in the Long Beach community who served as founding executive director at Long Beach Forward (LBF). She discussed her experience with the Building Healthy Communities Long Beach (BHCLB) project, an initiative through The California Endowment that led to the creation of LBF. Petit presented a photo taken a decade ago of tables of people reviewing drafts of a governance document for BHCLB. While the initiative also hosted outdoor community events, spent long evenings at city council meetings, and organized protests, she chose to highlight this image because it features people with different connections to the community working together. Three women sit in the forefront of the photo: one was a representative from the mayor's office, another was a community resident and leader, and the third was an organizational leader. Petit described LBF as the glue that brings together residents, community organizers, and decision makers, providing them with the tools and resources they need to create positive change. LBF supports community leaders and works to advance equitable policies. The organization operates from the belief that everyone in Long Beach should be able to influence the decisions that affect their lives, but often low-income communities of color are left out of decision-making processes.

The ability to influence decision-making processes can literally be a matter of life and death for Long Beach residents because there is a 7-year life expectancy disparity between zip codes in Long Beach, said Petit (City of Long Beach Department of Health and Human Services, 2013). She added that this gap expands when comparing census tract data, which reveals that the life expectancy for residents in whiter, wealthier zip codes is as much as 17 years longer than in areas largely comprising low-income people of color. LBF works to ensure that residents who are typically left out of decision making are heard on matters of environmental justice, economic inclusion, equity in education, and more. While advocates are not always understood or welcomed in city hall or at the school district, BHCLB and other initiatives have successfully changed more than 40 policies and practices in Long Beach, remarked Petit. This coalition of more than 50 organizations achieved these changes by shifting the narrative from exclusion to inclusion, highlighting systemic inequities, and uplifting the experiences of people most affected by these issues.

Singhal commented that the photo shows several people absorbed in thought and others engaged in animated conversation, which indicates it was a space where various groups and different voices could co-create moments of reflection and of conversation.

COMMUNITY-CENTERED REVITALIZATION

Michelle Carrillo, director of programs and community solutions at Humboldt Area Foundation, is from Del Norte County in northern California.[6] While this region has been *Mee-shvm-dvn*—or a place of plenty—for the Indigenous Tolowa people since the beginning of time, the community has also experienced great losses in the forms of genocide and a boom-and-bust economy over the past 150 years. However, the community members help one another in times of disaster, including during the current COVID-19 pandemic. Her predecessors had the forethought to collectively build a community founded in service for the benefit of future generations, said Carrillo. Reaching across arbitrary county and state lines, they have worked toward a vision of a thriving, just, healthy, and equitable region.

Carrillo described the area as a "small, predominantly white, rural, conservative community where the redwoods meet the sea," and it has

---

[6] More information about Humboldt Area Foundation is available at https://www.hafoundation.org (accessed March 7, 2021).

been a place of change, growth, and perseverance toward achieving a greater purpose. In 2011, Del Norte County ranked 55th out of 58 counties for health outcomes in the state of California (University of Wisconsin Population Health Institute, 2011). At that time, Carrillo was 22 years old and had just returned home from college to begin her career. The 2008 Great Recession was still affecting this rural community, and the perception that success could only be achieved by leaving the area was common. However, she saw returning to her home community as a path to a meaningful career and livelihood. Even while navigating life as a single working mother, she found deep connections with people who believed in her and invested in her development as a leader in systems change for health equity. That year, community leaders began a decade-long journey to build a healthy community by way of The California Endowment's Building Healthy Communities initiative.

At the start of the process, the notion that Del Norte could succeed in collaborating across party lines, systems, governments, and nations to address health equity seemed unlikely, said Carrillo. The vision of a community that fosters the dreams of every child sounded radical and unattainable; nonetheless, the work was carried forward. Setting universal goals around literacy, food access, and other critical intervention points, the coalition adopted an empathetic lens in understanding the barriers and systematic oppression many community members were experiencing. They created space to reimagine the future and to co-design solutions to realize envisioned possibilities. Today, Del Norte is ranked 45th out of 58 counties for health outcomes in the state (University of Wisconsin Population Health Institute, 2020). Carrillo said her community has achieved progress by shifting the way people think about themselves, their neighbors, their community, and their future. Singhal remarked on the value of acknowledging predecessors, creating spaces, holding conversations, and drawing upon personal narratives.

DISCUSSSION

Personal Impact of Community Power

Gunderson asked the panelists what they have learned about themselves and about community power building from the communities they serve. Referencing Carrillo's narrative of returning home and being blessed by her community, Gunderson posited that communities trust leaders seen as being transformed by their membership in the community. He asked about the personal effect the power of community has had on the panelists.

Ferdinand responded that Gunderson's statements are consistent with the empowerment narrative of the Sankofa organization. Rather than viewing the organization as empowering others, the staff at Sankofa see the organization as part of an ecosystem in which everyone is working and learning together. This enables Sankofa staff to understand the wisdom of the community members with whom they work. They are able to understand the importance of the work beyond the confines of studies, theories, or public health datasets. People at Sankofa are themselves transformed because they operate at the ground level to create work that the community relates to, said Ferdinand. The work is centralized around collaboration, not merely based on preset concepts of Sankofa's identity and agenda. The organization uses a community health ambassador model, in which community members, leaders, and other stakeholders formulate programs, plan systems, and make decisions for future efforts. This type of communal decision making creates transparent approaches that foster project sustainability, Ferdinand stated. When work belongs to the larger community, power and space are created to facilitate it. This signifies the difference between holding onto power and building power with one another. Singhal commented that this perspective of leadership looks beyond "Who am I?" to "Whose am I?"

Llanes Pulido remarked that she has learned to pay attention to what is said explicitly and what is omitted. Power dynamics and systems of oppression should be discussed explicitly in conversations about power, she contended. She shared GAVA's origins as an initiative before its independent incorporation. Inspired efforts funded by The California Endowment (TCE) and increasing statistical findings nationwide indicating that zip codes are better predictors of health outcomes than genetic codes, the Michael & Susan Dell Foundation catalyzed a 5-year, place-based childhood obesity intervention. Llanes Pulido recalled constructive critique from an equity specialist who grew up in Dove Springs, a neighborhood in southeast Austin at the center of GAVA's work. This colleague asked the initiative's catalyst funders, "When you say, 'zip codes,' what are you *not* saying?" and followed this with additional questions about the commonalities among people living in those zip codes and the reasons why they live there. Aliya Hussaini, the lead catalyst program officer, knew from her practice as a pediatrician that to be effective, the initiative would have to move beyond trying to influence individual behaviors, and look at community access to the resources people need to take care of themselves in a healthy manner. Llanes Pulido said the funders were curious and flexible in allowing the project to adapt to community needs, but they still ran against constraints and found tension among partners with each shift in addressing root causes.

A few years later, GAVA became an independent organization and began explicitly talking about power and antiracism in an intersectional way. This created space to discuss neighborhood stability and climate resilience as essential lenses in driving longitudinal health outcomes and the associated long-term sustainability of communities. Llanes Pulido said short- and intermediate-term health initiatives are of limited value if people continue to be exposed to forces that are negatively affecting them, or if they are displayed from the communities that support their health. This shift in focus made it more difficult to secure funding as a place-based health initiative among traditional funders of childhood health, she noted. However, by using creativity, community organizing, and collaborative strategic planning, the organization worked to galvanize power not only across residents, but also across institutional partners and philanthropic funders taking the lead from frontline communities addressing health equity.

Singhal remarked that Bobby Milstein, director of systems strategy at ReThink Health, often says that growth takes place in the direction of the questions asked, which not only involves asking the right questions, but also being aware of what is not being asked.

Sostaita emphasized the importance of listening to the needs of the people. He offered an example from ICSF's early days when traffic stops (checkpoints) deterred immigrants from coming to church. Police would stop people in their neighborhoods who lacked driver's licenses because of their undocumented status. ICSF partnered with several organizations to encourage the police department to move the checkpoints. Sostaita added that relationships can create a strong community. In another example, the police department shortened the amount of time in which one could apply for a U visa (abuse or violence), which caused some people to lose the possibility of resolving their immigration status. Through a relationship with the chief of police, ICSF, along with the North Carolina Latino Congress, successfully advocated for the time period in which one could apply for a visa to be extended to 5 years. He commented that many people are on the "dark side," and he works to build bridges to bring them to the light. Sostaita said this work has changed him, because he has come to share in the needs and sadness of the people with whom he works.

Petit said that she has been transformed by this work through watching people who have lived in Long Beach their entire lives begin to understand how power moves and how decisions are made in their community. As they learn how to organize to affect decision making, they found their power. She described being particularly inspired by youth organizing, as the lessons these young people are learning will stay with them throughout their lives. These efforts shift the narrative from an expectation that the status quo will remain in place to people using their voices for change. Furthermore, health can be a through line for discussing inequities. Redlining policies and other racist practices led to zip code–related health inequities, said Petit.[7] She noted these issues extend beyond Long Beach to the nation at large. LBF has worked to be more explicit about race and class, and it organizes around a vision in which race, class, and income do not determine one's future in Long Beach.

Carrillo remarked that centering race in this work has been an evolving process, especially in her area of northern California, where many people do not acknowledge the continued relevance of race. While inequities exist, systems have been built to mask them, she said. Traditional community engagement can be transactional, with quantifiable goals created around event attendance and survey completion. Community engagement becomes meaningful when power is discussed and listening is prioritized. For instance, organizers seeking to help children develop literacy skills can visit with mothers in their homes on the tribal reservation, learning about the daily lived experiences of the mothers and their children. The organizers and mothers can then co-design solutions together. Rather than approaching mothers with interventions, Carillo added, this work involves acknowledging the barriers built by an entire system of oppression, including lack of access to preschool, healthy food, and transportation. Having resources in place enables people to make decisions for their children that foster success.

Power as Health

Gunderson suggested that power can expand beyond working toward health to being an embodiment of health in and of itself. For instance, empowered communities may be more likely to mobilize vaccination efforts. He posited that this expression of agency and the energy it generates are healthy, and he asked Ferdinand to comment on this concept of "power as health." Ferdinand responded that Sankofa has made health the core aspect of its programming and approach to the work, because people may not perceive themselves and their health as primary. For instance, in moving through daily activities, people may not pause to consider factors that are affecting their quality of life, longevity, and propensity to become chronically ill, as well as leading to disparities that affect health outcomes. Health is core to all those aspects, and one's quality of health is contingent on access issues, said Ferdinand. This includes access to tangible items like healthy foods, as well as more abstract elements, such as a safe, stable living environment. Living situations involving stressors and trauma not

---

[7] Redlining is a discriminatory practice in which financial services such as mortgages, insurance, and loans are systematically denied based on race or ethnicity.

only affect biometric health, but they also affect social and mental health, parenting decisions, and family and community dynamics.

The Sankofa organization originally focused on food and community, noted Ferdinand. In 2008, only a few years after the community was devastated by Hurricane Katrina, the organization's initial project was a monthly marketplace. The creation of a venue for people to gather and engage with one another while buying fresh produce was rooted in an acknowledgment that healthy behavior extends beyond diet. The act of communing with one another and exchanging stories and love with neighbors can generate hope and yield health benefits, said Ferdinand. Environment also plays a role in health and community. To this end, Sankofa is involved in a project in which 40 acres of underresourced, neglected green space is being transformed into a community wetland park. Additionally, a commercial space in the neighborhood will be repurposed into a Fresh Stop market that will sell fresh produce and feature a learning kitchen for the community. Other opportunities for community revitalization are enabling residents to develop and own their own businesses. Ferdinand remarked that a variety of approaches to supporting health outcomes can be used. For example, transforming vacant, blighted land into commercially viable space and enabling people to learn and develop business skill sets can simultaneously support their health.

Gunderson added that public health and health care commonly refer to communities such Ferdinand's as "underserved," with the implication being that they have not received adequate services. He suggested that the way she discusses her community might better be described as "underliberated." Rather than needing additional services, communities need governments and institutions to remove the barriers that impose challenges to communities' ability to solve their own problems. Gunderson asked Ferdinand to discuss *served* versus *liberated* language. She replied that she does not use the term *underserved*, and prefers to describe the lack of equitable resources in her community as *underresourced*. Long-neglected, large disparities exist in the resources her community can access compared with those available in other parts of New Orleans, said Ferdinand.

Role of State Funding in Community Building

A participant working in a state health department asked for advice in funding place-based initiatives in communities working to use state-level power and federal funding streams to improve health equity and reduce health disparities. The participant asked how to leverage the power of a state health department to shift the flow of funding to the community without assuming a domineering role or violating community trust. Gunderson asked the panelists for examples of state departments providing assistance without inadvertently hurting the communities in these efforts.

Carrillo replied that time and resources should be invested in deep listening with the community, for the community will generate solutions if given the space to do so. Institutions that approach the community with favored solutions and action items miss an opportunity to build trust and achieve the level of change that comes with community-generated problem identification and solutions. Many communities have repeated experience with this type of process—one that is done "to" communities rather than done "with" them—especially in rural and tribal areas. Furthermore, while access to data is at play, it is rarely talked about, she noted. Communities such as hers are often undercounted in the U.S. census and in data for funding, a process that can lead to community invisibility. In addition to improved quantitative data, qualitative data in which communities describe what is happening in their neighborhoods should be collected, advised Carrillo. Increased spending is required to collect the quantitative and qualitative data needed to understand the dynamics of a small community.

Petit stated that LBF has engaged with government partnerships in different ways, albeit with varying results. She advised that institutions relinquish control of structuring the process of addressing health inequities. Rather than acting as core leader, the funding institution should partner with organizations who are connected to communities at a grassroots level. Often the structure of government lends itself to working with one large organization or statewide body, but that approach does not result in resources reaching communities that are experiencing the deepest health inequities, said Petit. Instead, creative models are needed that funnel resources directly to communities and allow them to define success. As government is often the target of power-building change efforts, this approach can be challenging for government institutions, she acknowledged. However, a focus on policy and systems change is important in transforming health inequities.

Sostaita recalled a health screening conducted at his church in which an older man's cholesterol and blood sugar readings were so high they called an ambulance. Afterward, Sostaita talked with the doctor performing the screenings and he voiced his concern that there may be many other people who are unaware they have high cholesterol or blood sugar. In building relationships with the local hospitals and the health department, Sostaita learned that the county health department had many resources available, but all were in English. He now offers weekly life-coaching classes to help community members seek out the resources they need, including the on-site health services he has organized, such as flu vaccines provided free of charge. Quoting Bible verse Matthew 7:7, "Ask and it will be given to you; seek and you will find; knock and the door will be opened to you," Sostaita said that if a person knocks, God will help. The partnerships health care providers have with the community are avenues for this help. Gunderson added that Sostaita is often "knocking on the hospital or public health door" on behalf of his community.

Llanes Pulido remarked that many decisions regarding health and education resources are not within municipal control in Texas. For instance, the city of Austin often attempts to enact policies that are considered progressive, but then receives backlash from the state. Proactive, grassroots organizing can interrupt this system by building and strengthening networks of people across Texas who are working toward the creation of just, healthy communities. She noted that the Texas corridor along Interstate 10 is experiencing the intersection of climate shocks and stressors—especially flooding and heat—as health equity issues. Politics can impede the efficient use of resources, and counties that collaborate with organizers are more likely to achieve gains during the COVID-19 pandemic, she suggested. Rural communities face additional challenges, given the comparative lack of nonprofit organizations in those areas. People in rural settings can begin organizing efforts by meeting in community centers, childcare centers, schools, churches, and with elders in the community to form a network.

Often, the very spaces for organizing and providing services to support health require protection, Llanes Pulido said. She recalled organizing in elementary schools about a decade ago regarding an unfunded state mandate to coordinate school health. While she worked to bring teachers and parents together in an effort to gain additional resources, massive teacher layoffs were taking place. Faculty were devastated that numerous colleagues were losing their jobs. In early 2020, her team had been working with childcare providers to ensure good nutrition and physical activities to benefit children's longitudinal health outcomes. They learned that the Texas health department created a new regulatory unit responsible for identifying unlicensed childcare providers. Llanes Pulido said the majority of childcare providers in the neighborhoods GAVA serves are unlicensed, and the regulation was perceived as a potential threat to the childcare ecosystem. She said that while the focus should be on making environments as healthy as possible, energy is required to protect childcare environments from being closed down and to plan for the disruption of childcare centers. She suggested that systems-level conversations be used to recalibrate funding models to reduce harm and address changing needs.

Community Health Metrics

A participant noted that not everything that counts is countable, and not everything that is countable counts. Singhal added that there is tremendous power in the determination of what is counted, and that with deep listening, that power can come from the community. Llanes Pulido remarked that GAVA is in the middle of creating a community-driven evaluation framework. The organization's initial 5 years as a place-based childhood obesity intervention endowed them with a set of 5-year longitudinal public health studies conducted by the University of Texas Health Science Center. The studies measured accessibility of healthy food and physical activity, utilization of community assets, health behaviors, and community readiness to address barriers to those resources. Llanes Pulido said that, while health behaviors improved and body mass index stabilized in adults with high exposure to GAVA's efforts, troubling evidence emerged regarding the child body mass index readings being measured. It also became clear that there were omitted variables. For example, during the research period there was an increase in economic stressors and two catastrophic floods that impacted the area, yet these were not addressed or evaluated in the study.

To account for a broader range of variables, GAVA is developing a community-driven set of evaluation indicators around health, demographics, and the environment. Working with colleagues at the Lyndon B. Johnson School of Public Affairs at The University of Texas, GAVA is determining how survey data on those areas can be collected, both through randomized samples and from the people who live in the communities GAVA serves with various levels of exposure to GAVA's community-based efforts. These data will then be used for multiple regression analysis to identify relationships among these interconnected variables. Carrillo added that the community is best equipped to determine the problems to address and goals to set; therefore, a community-driven approach is needed in determining metrics and learning focus areas. Furthermore, community input should be used to identify factors contributing to a desired outcome that is not yet being achieved as well as the changes required to arrive at a desired outcome. She described this process as continually evolving (it is an iterative process that deepens with relationship and trust over time).

Direction of Power

A participant noted that the U.S. federal government's response to the COVID-19 pandemic is often characterized as being insufficient, ineffective, or inconsistent, which suggests that a stronger top-down approach is needed. Singhal asked if the reverse might be true—that the problem lies in communities being neither adequately resourced nor trusted to develop their own responses to the pandemic. Carrillo said this is not an either/or situation, but rather a both/and situation. The needed change requires everyone to step into the power they have, and one cannot deny that the federal government has power. Power and responsibility exist at all levels, from grassroots communities to the federal government. She said that the focus should be placed on leveraging power at each level and working together across levels.

Llanes Pulido commented on assumptions that neighborhood stability and social cohesion support people's health and their ability to withstand disaster. GAVA wants to further explore and challenge those assumptions. For instance, it is examining how the racial background of people living in the same zip code affects the perceptions of safety in regard to police interactions. This example represents a number of varying factors at the intersection of healthy food, physical activity, and neighborhood stability. An understanding that the people who experience effects are key to creating solutions has developed in the field of health equity, said Llanes Pulido. Allowing communities to lead conversations enables them to identify the underlying problems that organizations should be focusing on.

Notable Community Features

Gunderson suggested that as community organizers, the panelists are likely to be less focused on the quantitative measurements of indicators than on a systematic observation of factors. He asked the panelists what factors they pay attention to when visiting a community. Petit replied that she is interested in experiencing different neighborhoods and noticing who lives in them and what types of jobs they have. While giving some visiting sociologists a tour of Long Beach, she took them to the wealthy neighborhood of Naples in order to compare the 2.65 percent unemployment rate of that community to the 19 percent joblessness rate in central Long Beach. When people advise others to live in certain parts of town versus others, there is a story behind that, said Petit. She is interested in the story of what a neighborhood feels like, the history behind why groups of people live there, and why there are dividing lines between parts of town. Petit added that environmental health collaboratives have organized "toxic tours" that highlight the environmental and health problems created by the pollution from Long Beach's large shipping port, oil refineries, and other aspects of the built environment.

Carrillo remarked that a tour of her community in northern California would involve both a bus and a boat. She would take visitors by bus to different community centers, garden spaces, and other places where people have created growth in vitality. The tour would also include neighborhoods affected by disinvestment to compare these to the possibilities seen in the growth communities. Next, there would be a 45-minute boat trip up the Klamath River to visit the Upper Yurok Reservation. While a state highway connects to the reservation, there are sections that are still a one-lane road along a cliff. She noted that the school received access to electricity via a generator only 2 years ago. The level of disconnection and disinvestment from institutions is readily apparent in this area, said Carrillo. This is powerful, juxtaposed to the richness and vitality of the people, community, and natural landscape of the region.

Singhal said he would take visitors to the parking lot of the Walmart in El Paso where 22 people were killed in the shooting that took place on August 3, 2019. A Grand Candela (grand candle) Memorial has been erected at the site. Made up of 22 arcs to symbolize the victims who lost their lives, the structure emits light that traverses across the U.S.-Mexico border and is visible to all.

Power-Building Imagery

Gunderson recounted a visit to a group within the Cesar Chavez ecology of organizations. *Chicanos Por La Causa* is a community-based organization in Phoenix, Arizona, that began with union organizing efforts around outlawing the short-handled hoe. Farm workers organized to ban this tool that required the user to bend over, leading to chronic back pain and long-term health issues. The image of the short-handled hoe serves as a powerful reminder of the difficult circumstances previous generations of organizers have faced and puts current challenges in perspective, said Gunderson. He asked the panelists about images that symbolize the uphill battles that those who came before them have faced.

Llanes Pulido is a second-generation organizer who grew up during the galvanizing phase of the environmental justice movement. In 1992, low-income communities of color with a budget of approximately $2,000 were able to successfully organize efforts resulting in six transnational oil companies vacating a fuel storage facility in East Austin. She said that the struggle involved in this successful effort gives her a sense of solidarity with Nigerian activists protesting Shell Oil. Llanes Pulido repeatedly reminds herself that her work in politics and organizing is made possible by the elders and ancestors who blazed a trail before her.

Carrillo shared a drawing created in 2009 to represent a vision of opportunities for young people to have meaningful work and connection to community. It featured a girl wearing a t-shirt that says, "I love this place because I can make it great." In one hand, she holds a toolbox containing research, writing, policy, advocacy, media, and public speaking. In her other hand, she holds a plan that includes education, a healthy lifestyle, economic security, hopes and dreams, and a community where she can find a job she loves and a healthy place to raise a family. Carrillo noted that when this drawing was created, it seemed an impossible dream. However, 12 years later, she is working with young people who are the embodiment of this vision. For example, a transgender youth hosted a county commissioner town hall and created a radio program about racial equity with the mayor in a rural, conservative community. In addition, a 22-year-old is serving on the city council. Carrillo grew up hearing that success necessitated leaving the community, but now young people have hopes and dreams within the community.

Petit held up a large paper circle with a heart on one side and an angry face emoji on the other. About 10 years ago, she and other activists were watching the mayor's annual State of the City address with frustration that much of what he said undercut the work they were doing. They decided to create a People's State of the City forum for presenting information to the community that politicians omit. This annual event now attracts as many as 500 attendees from the community. Participants are given the circles as a tool to express how they feel about the information that is presented. She said the two-sided circle represents her community's ability to definite its own narrative and priorities.

Sostaita said his dream is always to bring the community together. Regardless of whether people are members of his church, he views all neighbors as his community. He noted that many young people feel lost and unsure of what to do. His church works to bring families and individuals together into community, a place where people can experience the power of education, health, hope, and healing.

Ferdinand held up a photograph of her father and uncle standing in front of the house they grew up in. She described the house as a place she loved, charming with its cobblestone driveway and rose bushes. The neighborhood was devastated by the floods of Hurricane Katrina, and the house is no longer there. The current condition of the neighborhood, with more vacant lots than homes, is difficult to reconcile with the lovely image in the photo, said Ferdinand. In spite of that, seeing the photo and remembering how much love her father and uncle had for their childhood home gives her hope in working to create a stronger community. She also presented a photo of Wetland Park, which is across the street from the neighborhood where her father spent his childhood. The park features beautiful water and wildlife, and children play there. In spite of its proximity to homes, alligators, coyotes, rabbits, and other animals and plants are flourishing there. Ferdinand said the creation of a space that simultaneously holds memories of ancestors and provides children with a place to explore, enjoy nature, and be free gives her hope.

Gunderson showed a painting that depicts a sun shining over places of worship from various religions. He stated that people come to worship in order to humble themselves before what they understand to be the ultimate power, and they leave places of worship ready to give of themselves in creating the future. The painting also depicts science, a field that continually provides new tools to use in imagining possibilities for our communities. Thus, this painting is a picture of power for him.

7

Amplifying the Empirical Base Linking Community Power and Health Equity

---

CHAPTER HIGHLIGHTS

- Three characteristics of power are pertinent to understanding community power: source, nature, and instruments. (Speer)
- Organizational practices to generate community power are dynamic, influenced by local community context, and they require additional research to be better understood in creating power-building outcomes. (Speer, Wright)
- Power building is not only a means to achieving health equity, it is an end in and of itself. (Martinez)
- Traditional research methods are not adequate to generate evidence of effective community-building practices, and responsive, immersive methods that capture variation in community-building practices are needed. (Cutts, Wright)
- Iterative learning cycles allow metrics to continually refine processes, programs, and policy. (Cutts, Parajón)
- Relational and contextual components are central to effective power-building practices. (Cutts, Martinez, Parajón, Speer, Wright)

The final session of the workshop explored how evidence can be used in improving community-building practices, policy, and funding decisions. Because power building is a complex, dynamic enterprise involving local control, new methods of generating evidence are needed to assess and inform practice. Panelists discussed the limitations of traditional research methods in evaluating power building, provided case studies of responsive assessment approaches, and outlined the work needed to create more effective community-building research tools. Hanh Cao Yu, chief learning officer at The California Endowment (TCE), moderated the session.

Yu remarked on the need to support community power efforts to achieve racial and health equity; this work should be guided by humility. Research and theory linking community power and health equity is nascent and largely conceptual, rather than empirical. Funders can build long-term, sustainable power infrastructures to support the work of communities by increasing investment and improving partnerships, said Yu. At the same time, strengthening the empirical evidence base linking health equity with community power can facilitate insights that can be applied to knowledge, practice, and power-building research.

PERSONAL DRIVE FOR POWER BUILDING

Yu asked each panelist to speak about his or her passion around community power. Paul Speer, professor and chair of the Department of Human and Organizational Development at Vanderbilt University, replied that he works to address the injustices taking place around the world by understanding community power and supporting groups that are developing and exercising it. Tia Martinez, chief executive officer at ForwardChange, said that her work is rooted in making meaning of the suffering and survival of her family and community. Using an analysis of power to make sense of the unequal distribution of suffering can help to unlock that dynamic and begin the healing process, she suggested.

Bill Wright, executive director at the Providence Health System Center for Outcomes Research and Education, remarked that systems change is too rare. Even with recognition that a system is not working for all people, it is common to address barriers by creating programs or altering an aspect of how people move through the system, rather than considering that the system itself may not be adequately adaptive to meet the needs of the people it is designed to serve. A systems change approach involves asking fundamental questions about how systems should be designed and about who should determine that design. Too often, service gaps are defined as "systems failures," when in actuality, some systems were designed to exclude specific populations, said Wright. In such cases, the system is functioning according to its original design. He added that regardless of the intentions under which a system was designed, attention should be given to identifying people that ought to have a role in designing the system. Power-building work embraces asking fundamental questions about how systems are constructed.

Teresa Cutts, professor at the Wake Forest School of Medicine's Public Health Sciences Division, recounted growing up in the Mississippi Delta in a community facing deep poverty. The hard-working people in her community lacked power, money, status, and higher education. She was born in a clinic approximately 500 feet from the burial site of civil rights activist Fanny Lou Hamer. Cutts recalled the unkindness, hatred, and abuse faced by African American children integrated into her community's schools during her childhood. She said she strives to undo some of that harm by offering kindness, respect, and humility. Her grandmother owned a dry goods store in a predominantly African American part of town, and Cutts helped in the store every Saturday throughout her childhood. She noted that this was an unusual experience for a white child to have; it led her to develop a deep, abiding respect for African American culture, which is full of authenticity, warmth, kindness, and community power. Cutts also witnessed the abject poverty experienced by community members despite their working 6.5 days each week, their fingers swollen from picking cotton in the hot Delta fields. She described the community as having transcended these hardships and challenging existence through the joy they shared with one another. Cutts added that her grandfather was a sharecropper who faced difficulties that contributed to her desire to shift the power differential early in her life.

Laura Parajón, professor and executive director of the Office of Community Health at the University of New Mexico, said that love is a steadfast commitment to the well-being of others. Quoting American philosopher Cornel West, she said "Justice is what love looks like in public." She added that she is driven by love, service, and empowerment, with community power being an integral part of her motivation. Yu remarked that she came to the United States as a refugee from Vietnam and is emboldened in her work by the devastation of colonialization and the Vietnam War.

CHALLENGES AND TENSIONS IN THE EXERCISE OF COMMUNITY POWER: PRACTICE IMPLICATIONS FOR RESEARCH

Speer noted that his presentation draws from work performed with his colleagues from Vanderbilt University, Jyoti Gupta and Krista Haapanen, and with Hahrie Han, professor and director of the Stavros Niarchos Foundation (SNF) Agora Institute at Johns Hopkins University.

Features of Power and Community Change

Speer outlined three features of power pertinent to understanding community power: source, nature, and instruments. The source is the basis of power that is exercised, and it may take the form of people or money. The nature of power involves how power operates, whether this be in a cooperative or conflictual fashion. Instruments of power are the mechanisms through which power is expressed. These include reward, punishment, and the ability to shape awareness and public debate. Minimally, community power requires developing a source of power, an understanding of how power works, and strategies through which to exercise it, said Speer.

A focus on power should be coupled with community change, or the ultimate effect of exercised power, said Speer. Change resulting from the exercise of power can take three forms: symbolic, incremental, and restructuring. Symbolic change involves a shift in outward appearance with stability in behavior. For instance, a person who trades their red shirts for blue ones, but does not alter any other behaviors, would exhibit symbolic change. Interventions resulting in symbolic change do not increase a community's resources.

In contrast, incremental change does involve an increase in valued resources, yet the overall distribution of a valued resource between the "haves" and "have-nots" remains stable. For example, in the 1960s the children's program Sesame Street was designed to address the gap in school readiness between impoverished and middle-class children (Ball and Bogatz, 1970). Intended to improve children's recognition of letters, words, colors, and numbers, Sesame Street increased school readiness for low-income children. However, middle-class children also watched it and improved their capacities, said Speer. Thus, this intervention increased a valued resource for both low- and middle-income children, but given the persisting school readiness gap, it did not change the overall distribution of resources. The third form of change is restructuring change, in which a shift in the distribution of a valued resource does take place. Speer noted that a restructuring change occurred with tax policy that has redistributed wealth in the United States since the late 1970s. In this case, a smaller number of people have a greater amount of wealth; thus, the restructuring change has created greater inequity. He and others working in the field of health equity are working toward more evenness in the allocation of resources, said Speer. Some research, Speer stated, focuses on individual behavior change as the outcome of interest and does not focus on systemic change. Behavior change generates symbolic or incremental change. In contrast, research indicates that systemic change with a focus on health equity generates access to better health and greater equity across populations, resulting in restructuring change. Therefore, advancing health equity requires altering the distribution of valued resources, and altering this distribution requires exercising community power, Speer commented.

Diversity and Dynamics of Power-Building Practices

In determining how local community-organizing groups can best build and develop power, Speer and his colleagues examine the activities or processes groups use to generate community power and the outcomes of these efforts. Overlaying this information with understandings of the dimensions of power and the forms of change results in a complex framework that indicates a high level of nuance in community interventions. Speer called for greater research attention to the complex processes that local community-building efforts engage in. He presented an overview of various dimensions and examples of community-based practice; these processes for developing community power include a wide range of strategies, tactics, and orientations (see Table 7-1). Studies can be shaped to capture these diverse power-building practices in order to draw distinctions and learn what is most effective, said Speer. He continued that critical differences in tactics, locus of intervention, and other key dimensions of community-based practice must be conceptualized and measured.

Adding to the complexity of power building, the implementation of any given practice is not static. The local community context—including the internal developmental goals of the organization—drives implementation. For instance, some organizations tend to participate in staff-driven decision making, while other groups engage in participatory leadership. Most groups do not fall singularly into one category or the other; rather, a tension and dialectic are present. At different points in time for various external reasons staff or local leaders may take a larger role. To understand how power is built, developed, and exercised, attention must be given to the practices taking place on the ground, said Speer. The tensions and dilemmas inherent in community dynamics can drive strategic decisions, and research in this area can inform best practices for building community power.

Implications for Community Power Research

Speer noted several implications for community power research. First, measurement of community power-building processes should be a priority for researchers. He provided an example that charted the distribution of staff organizers meeting with community members in groups of various sizes. Some organizations focus on small meetings held with one or two individuals at a time, while other groups work to develop a broader range of relationships through meeting with small groups. He added that the distributions of meeting size can affect the outcomes of building power. Second, a greater focus on the relational qualities of both power building and community change is needed, he recommended.

TABLE 7-1 Diverse Practices for Developing Community Power

Dimensions	Descriptions/Common Alternatives
Source of problems	• Problems arise from deficits of people or lack of skills and/or motivation • Problems arise from conditions of environment • Problems arise from systems of exploitation and the powerlessness they produce
Change strategies	• People solve their own problems rather than looking to institutions to solve their problems for them • Communities seek experts to address problems; need for technocratic solutions • People form collective power and demand changes
Change tactics	• Consensus building, better communication, educate people, social marketing • Seek others—experts, elected officials, hierarchical figures—and through respect, kindness, and appreciation relinquish community responsibilities to elites • Confront those with power about hypocrisy on values, stated claims, democratic principles; conflict and direct action when necessary; negotiate with power to achieve outcomes
Orientation to power structure	• Collaborators and partners in common goals • Employers, sponsors, meritorious elites • Actors external to community with divergent interests from residents
Boundary definitions	• Target geographic area • Target relational communities • Target identity-based alignments (gender, race, ability, class) • Target existing group memberships (school, faith group, workplace)
Role of organizer	• Teacher, catalyst, booster, problem solver, broker, planner, analyst, expert, program implementer, activist, advocate, agitator, partisan, negotiator
Locus of intervention	• Point of production—site of exploitation (strikes, pickets, slowdowns) • Point of consumption—visible endpoint of exploitation (boycotts, demonstrations) • Point of destruction—where there is harm (strip mine, landfill) • Point of decision—site where elites determine policies (board meeting, slumlord office) • Point of assumption—challenges unreflected-upon beliefs
Outcomes valued	• Expressive action—focus on communicating values, culture, or emotions • Valued instrumental actions—focus on tangible change and achieving goals

SOURCE: Adapted from Speer presentation, January 29, 2021.

For instance, the distribution of young to middle-aged men in the community has a curvilinear relationship to violent crime, where the higher proportion of young to middle-aged men is associated with more violent crime in the community. Thus, relational qualities (in this example, intergenerational relationships) can be critical to power-building and change efforts, said Speer. Third, research methods that examine longitudinal and multilevel relationships are key, he stated. Such research enables comparisons to be made among the same group over time and with other groups, providing a basis for determining the effectiveness of change efforts.

Speer added that organizational practices to generate community power are not fixed processes. They are dynamic processes that are influenced by local community context and require additional research to be better understood in creating power-building outcomes.

THE CALIFORNIA ENDOWMENT: BUILDING HEALTHY COMMUNITIES

Martinez discussed the evolution of TCE's Building Healthy Communities (BHC) project over the span of a decade. While many place-based programs focus on service saturation, such as the Harlem Children's Zone, BHC targeted power building and policy and systems change in 14 neighborhoods. The BHC theory of change proposes that building power leads residents to push for policy and systems change, which in turn improves the opportunity environment. Over time, the improved opportunity environment affects social determinants of health, eventually resulting in a change in population-level health status.

Presenting a timeline of BHC initiatives from 2010 through 2019 at the various neighborhood sites, Martinez highlighted the substantial amount of innovative experimentation conducted by BHC grantees and TCE leadership and program managers. The rapid rate at which TCE learns and adapts can be challenging to keep pace with, but its processes are focused on delivering outcomes. In 2010, the BHC framework was structured around the "big four results:" (1) to provide a healthy home for all children, (2) to reverse the childhood obesity epidemic, (3) to increase school attendance, and (4) to reduce youth violence. As BHC progressed, change drivers such as people power, youth leadership, narrative change, and policy innovation emerged, leading to the development of the BHC theory of change in 2013.

Lessons Learned in Centering Grassroots Power Building

Over the next several years, BHC shifted its focus and practices in response to an evolving understanding of power building. While continuing to use multiple approaches and methods in policy advocacy and legal efforts, the foundation determined that grassroots power building must be placed at the center its efforts, said Martinez. Furthermore, grassroots efforts for racial justice were made primary. Originally, the mission for the project was "health equity equals health justice for all." With the shift toward power building and racial justice efforts, the mission evolved to "building voice and power for a healthy and inclusive California." Internal power was realigned from prioritizing funder "grasstops" leadership to prioritizing grassroots leadership. Martinez noted a midpoint evaluation conducted by the University of Southern California Program for Environmental and Regional Equity (USC PERE) was instrumental in BHC's pivot. This evaluation found that:

> During the first half of BHC, an emphasis has been on … achieving health equity through professional advocacy and communications efforts bolstered by community voice and mobilization…. The health equity equation should lead with community organizing, leadership development, and grassroots advocacy—and then bolster those efforts with professional advocacy and communications. (Ito and Pastor, 2018)

The recalibration of BHC's focus elevated power building from a secondary instrumental driver—a method to achieve health equity—to a primary driver and ultimately an end in itself, she added.

Lesson 1: Evolve the Definition of "People Power"

Martinez stated that when BHC began, the working definition of "people power" was resident engagement. In this model, the residents affected by an issue provide input, bolster public debate, and influence policy decisions. The role of the community is to draw attendance to events such as board meetings and city council meetings. This method views power as the aggregation of many individuals' efforts, and thereby more people speaking at an event equates to more power. When the project got underway in 2009–2010, BHC worked from this construct and viewed the foundation as responsible for setting results and desired outcomes and then soliciting feedback from the community on how to achieve those preset goals.

The foundation quickly realized that power exercised by community is more complex and nuanced than its original understanding, said Martinez. During the period from 2011 to 2015—the early implementation phase of BHC—the definition of "people power" shifted from resident engagement to resident agency. Instead of a conglomeration of individuals speaking at an event, this framework views the role of residents as collectively collaborating to shape campaigns and programs to proactively demand a response from policy makers and system leaders. This construct implies the need for strong organizations that are responsible for recruiting members and developing their skill sets, creating policy agendas, and exercising power. The role of community then pivots from residents providing input to organizations possessing agency. Rather than independently setting goals, the foundation brings together grassroots organizations, service organizations, and system leaders to collaboratively build solutions.

During BHC's midpoint review phase (2016–2018), the definition of "people power" once again shifted, this time to a "seeds of people power" understanding. This approach expands beyond community members shaping campaigns to community-led initiatives gaining traction and flexing their leadership in the strategy process, determining the issues to focus on and the approaches to use in addressing them. Martinez remarked that at this stage, community organizations did away with goals set by TCE and created their own path forward. For instance, community organizations decided to move their work in schools away from a focus on truancy prevention to healing justice efforts. In this iteration, BHC shifted from bringing community partners to the table to becoming a node for resident-led formations to connect, build relationships, and access resources for growth.

The final evolution of BHC's working definition of "people power" came in 2019 with the transition planning phase. Martinez explained that this construct involves a power-building ecosystem in which diverse community-led initiatives align toward greater mutuality and complementarity while centering grassroots organizing for racial justice. In this framework, the roles of residents, the community, and the foundation are encompassed within the ecosystem.

Lesson 2: Building Power Requires an Ecosystem

The ecosystem model centers grassroots groups supported by a robust network of allies from diverse disciplines (see Figure 7-1). USC PERE described this ecosystem:

> Organizing and base building alone are insufficient to influence those who have the authority, resources, and power to make the kinds of decisions that will improve the lives of historically excluded people and reduce inequities.... A broader ecosystem of organizations with diverse capacities, skills, and expertise—and with reach from the local to regional to the state levels—is required to get to the big goal of health and justice for all. (USC PERE, 2018)

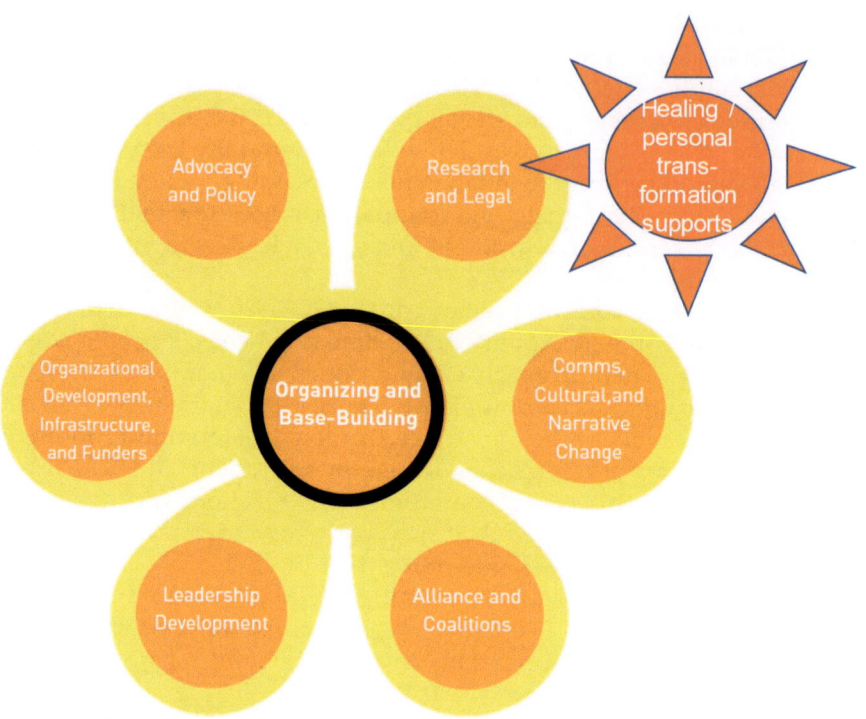

FIGURE 7-1 Power-building ecosystem.
SOURCES: Martinez presentation, January 29, 2021; USC PERE, 2018.

Martinez emphasized that this framework continues to feature advocacy, research, and leadership development as necessary components, but they are ancillary to the centralized element of organizing groups and helping them to build up their base.

Lesson 3: The Crucial Role of Healing in Social Movement Work

After the power-building ecosystem model was developed, BHC identified healing and personal transformation supports as a missing component, said Martinez. Through ongoing communication between BHC program managers and grantees, BHC established that structural change through power building is always imperative, but removing or reforming harmful structures will not automatically undo the psychological, spiritual, and physical damage done to bodies, souls, and minds over generations. Structural change will not address the internal wounds already inflicted on people by systems, history, and each other. Without attention to healing, organizers, advocates, and community members can turn on one another or turn on themselves and self-destruct, continued Martinez. Rage can motivate people, but it can also become destructive and undermine the movement if directed at colleagues and allies. By proactively addressing past and current wounds, building a health-centered movement enables those most affected—and hence the most hurt by—oppressive systems to fully participate as advocates and leaders in the movement, while at the same time building the critical consciousness needed to interpret the world and act to transform it.

Lesson 4: Putting Narrative Strategy in Service of Grassroots Power Building

As BHC processes shifted to allow communities to have agency, strategy around narrative change also transformed. Initially using a traditional strategy, TCE led the effort to change social norms and partnered with big media consulting firms in this work. Martinez noted that with deeper understanding of power building, TCE learned that narrative change should be led by the community and deeply embedded in the greater grassroots power-building effort. Narrative change is not a communications strategy separate from power, but a part of power itself. An essential component of community organization, establishing narrative change is part of the power-building ecosystem. By pivoting from a top-down approach in which media firms direct narrative change strategy, BHC acknowledged the inherent power of historically marginalized communities developing their own cultural and narrative change strategies.

Lesson 5: Align Lessons with the Faces of Power Model

Martinez outlined the alignment of the lessons BHC learned with the Grassroots Policy Project's "three faces of power" model, which identifies: (1) the power to win demands, (2) the power to drive the agenda, and (3) the power to shape common sense. The power to win demands applies to BHC's focus on "people power" as the change engine. The power to drive the agenda relates to the understanding that building power requires more than strong organizations—it requires an ecosystem. The power to shape common sense pertains to putting narrative strategy in service of grassroots power building.

Rethinking the Funder Role

The lessons gleaned over the decade of BHC initiatives led TCE to rethink its role as a funder, said Martinez. To move away from a position of telling or leading organizations in their course of action—thereby having power over them—TCE has shifted to having power with the grantees in allowing the movement to lead. She stated that funders are not always transparent or consistent, vacillating from having too little involvement to being too heavily involved. To avoid this, TCE has created a feedback loop with grantees to listen to them and to adjust as necessary. This allows TCE to maintain a level of involvement that grantees value. Martinez remarked that funders often measure grantee success based on factors such as rapid response, highly visible policy wins, ability to leverage the insider track, and superficial metrics (e.g., numbers of residents attending events). Instead, TCE is shifting toward measuring success by assessing systems transformation that is deeply rooted in the most affected communities and in generational change, as well as developing new metrics for authentic power building. Lastly, the core competency of TCE program managers is their ability to pivot from strengthening individual organizations to learning how to cultivate a robust ecosystem for health-centered movements.

BUILDING EVIDENCE FOR POWER AND HEALTH: THE BHC INITIATIVE AS A LEARNING ENGINE

Using the BHC initiative as a case study, Wright outlined the challenges faced in generating evidence of the efficacy of power building, as well as generating evidence of the work being done to address those challenges. Both the scope and nature of BHC make it difficult to evaluate the program using traditional methods. As an ecosystem of efforts, BHC involves $1.8 billion spread over more than 10,000 grants, with activities in 14 cities and complementary statewide work, all of which is centered on power building. Based on the concept that communities are best able to resolve their own key health challenges, BHC operates with a theory of change that sees power building as the key strategy for addressing health equity, Wright noted. Instead of investing in specific programs or services, the role of the initiative is to help those communities build the power needed to make changes in policies and systems that affect community health outcomes. Related activities and strategies are led by local partners, whose approaches are not prescribed.

Limitations of Traditional Evaluation Methods for Application to Power Building

This represents a fundamental shift in approaching community health, and the traditional scientific tool kit is ill equipped to generate evidence for this new approach, said Wright. The vast majority of scientific tools are used for inference, where attribution of effect is predicated on comparing variation across boundaries. Careful methods of defining boundaries—be they time intervals, groups, or other distinctions—are used to ensure that comparisons are fair. These range from fully randomized designs to observational studies involving case matching. In the context of BHC, typical studies might examine BHC sites and similar sites where BHC is not active to compare trends of key outcomes over time. These data then inform an evaluation of whether BHC "worked," Wright remarked. However, such methods rely on a degree of certainty about what happened on either side of the inference boundaries. He noted that a central feature of power-building initiatives is that researchers do not control what takes place. Instead, the boundaries, the approach to goals, and even the goals and strategies themselves are permeable by design and are ultimately determined by communities. Thus, different BHC communities may focus on different goals or strategies at various times.

For instance, any given body of work within the scope of BHC may be adopted by different BHC sites at various times and to varying degrees. For instance, site A may have focused on that work from the start, site B may have begun that work halfway through their grant period, and site C may have used an entirely different approach. Wright remarked that evaluating an intervention monolithically would bias findings toward the null by including factors on the treatment side of the inference boundary that actually belong on the comparison side. The importance of factoring in local context that Speer described is relevant to this example, Wright noted. In programmatic approaches, the "who, what, when, where, and how much" of interventions are typically known. In contrast, in the context of building power, the people on the ground in communities determine those factors; by design, researchers do not control them. Thus, the boundaries that are well defined in traditional research are permeable in power-building work. Boundaries of place are permeable because power, policy, and systems changes are not neatly contained by location. Boundaries of time are permeable, as described above and in communities that have long engaged in power building. The boundaries of who and what are permeable in the locally run nature of efforts tailored to each community.

Building Context-Rich Approaches to Power-Building Data

More thoughtful inference boundaries are needed to evaluate power-building initiatives, said Wright. Moving beyond a simple boundary—such as whether or not a location was a BHC site—a more granular approach can be used in identifying what happened, where it happened, how much of it happened, and who it happened with. Within a community power-building framework, decisions are made locally and emerge as the work progresses, signifying that context will vary across sites. Wright stated that scientists typically consider variation in an intervention as unwelcome noise. In a context-rich approach, variation is viewed as a source of strength and an engine for learning. Once methods of learning from variation are developed, elements of the traditional research tool kit can then be used, he noted.

To translate a data-rich approach to an empirical tool set, BHC begins with potential outcomes—for instance, disparities in school discipline rates—and then identifies related investments and activities that took place and indexes when they took place. Contexts in the community related to the specific issue are explored, and inference boundaries are then built around context-specific subsets of data. Time becomes a set of fixed intervals relative to index dates that represent when context-specific activities happened, explained Wright. Designs such as comparative interrupted time series can be used to assess and compare changes in the trends of key outcomes over time across inferential boundaries (see Figure 7-2). Thus, scientists can use familiar tools in a context-informed way.

Wright noted that this approach required the construction of an integrated mixed-methods engine to create a context-rich analytic environment. Much of the data needed for this type of approach comes from narrative reports, such as grant descriptions and grant reporting. BHC developed a method of collapsing narratives, coding them into discrete data that summarizes key aspects of the "who, what, when, where, and how much" of what took place in the community work. More structured

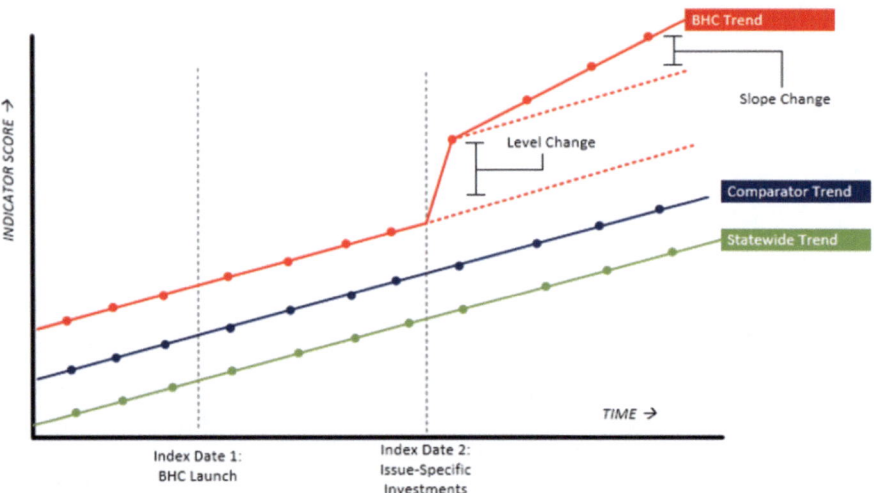

FIGURE 7-2 Example of comparative interrupted time series design.
SOURCE: Wright presentation, January 29, 2021.

outcome data from surveys and administrative datasets are collected for all relevant geographies and subgroups. A universal coding framework serves as connective tissue between the disparate elements of the data ecosystem. Every element of data—whether it is discrete data from a state dataset or survey or narrative data from a report or interview—is then coded and tagged with attributes. The attributes can include time, place, population, intended domain of effect, and any other factors that may link data points. Wright explained that for any given question, the elements most appropriate to the specific context can be selected from the data ecosystem. Elements may include BHC investments and activities, measures of power building, policy or systems change, and outcomes indicators. The universal coding framework enables data to be linked together in the context of the theory of change and allows for the production of outcomes models.

Overlaying the universal coding framework on the BHC theory of change facilitates understanding of direct and indirect effects of power building, Wright noted. Using this approach, one can determine how much variation in any given outcome over time can be attributed to various potential effect pathways, including power building. For instance, one can examine how much variation is associated with being a BHC site or how much variation is associated specifically with changes in power-building indicators. Moving through the stages of BHC's theory of change, every set of indicators can be positioned as an outcome or as a mediator/moderator; an indicator that is an outcome at one stage can become a potential mediator in the following stage. For any given BHC campaign, estimates can be produced by assessing how much variation is attributable to each potential effect pathway, thus elucidating the mechanisms that created change.

Creating Learning Architecture

Wright remarked that this approach moves beyond a pass/fail evaluation to create a system for learning. Tracing each point of the data overlaid on the theory of change, evidence will either support or fail to support the hypothesized relationship. In testing different effect pathways across the theory of change, patterns will emerge. These patterns will inevitably vary for different contexts and outcomes, which leads to learning, said Wright. The nuanced stories accompanying these patterns create enormous variation across the BHC ecosystem. Instead of treating variation like a bug, this approach uses variation as a feature in the creation of a rigorous learning architecture. The knowledge gained through the use of such learning architecture informs the role of power building in addressing health and equity, he noted.

To illustrate what this process looks like in practice, Wright provided an example from a BHC analysis. It began with a foundational question: Were BHC investments in resident organizing associated with more active, civically engaged communities over time? They coded all 10,615 BHC grants with the universal coding framework to capture the "who, what, when, where, and how much" of components in each grant. Next, they identified a set of potential indicators representing community engagement from various sources, such as voting records and community surveys. Then they tagged investments, activities, and contextual factors related to resident organizing, voting rights, community voice, and representation in positions of power. Creating a visual representation of how these elements may relate to one another, they plotted an analytic pathway connecting the areas of engagement. They then used the inference framework to build a series of multivariate models to test the responsiveness of the indicators to the power-building work over time. For instance, BHC examined whether resident engagement work improved voter turnout, an indicator of an active and engaged community. BHC determined that a $5 per capita investment was associated with a 0.38 percentage point increase in voting participation. Therefore, BHC was able to identify a dose–response relationship in investing in resident engagement and voter turnout.

Such knowledge has multiple applications, including helping TCE to develop and adapt its own strategy. The model's parameter estimates can be used to map out each community's strategy and to inform the field about efforts likely to result in desired outcomes. BHC is creating "impact profiles" to help TCE and others anticipate outcomes of a given level of investment or activity. These impact profiles are not performed one outcome at a time, as this work is not a transactional effort. Instead, they are conducted across an ecosystem of connected outcomes. In addition to informing strategy, this builds a case for the value of the work, said Wright.

Better understanding of the role of power building and the mechanisms by which desired outcomes are created bolsters confidence in investment in resident engagement activities. Wright outlined how the learning system can also be used to test each step of BHC's theory of change. The first step involves examining whether activities supported by BHC activities result in power building, as described in the voter turnout example. Next, the relationship between power building and policy and systems change is explored to determine whether an association exists between improvements in power-building indicators and adoption of key policy changes. Finally, the framework can be used to identify whether policy and systems changes do indeed result in different health outcomes. Wright noted that this is the direction toward which BHC's work is evolving.

The BHC theory of change represents a major shift from addressing health through programmatic response to power building within communities, said Wright. He contended that it is critical to move beyond assessing whether BHC improved outcomes to developing an understanding of how those improvements were created and who was affected. Such understanding enables the improvements to be sustained and expanded. Wright added that the more BHC can take advantage of the rich variation across BHC communities, the more BHC can serve as a data ecosystem for the field at large. This learning engine will then become a shared asset used by a community of thinkers and researchers who together can advance the state of science to support this work.

COMMUNITY POWER AND HEALTH EQUITY: THE MEMPHIS MODEL'S CARDIAC DISPARITY CASE STUDY

Cutts reviewed a case study in which the Congregational Health Network (CHN), a health system-faith community partnership, was able to decrease sudden cardiac deaths in African Americans within the course of 18 months.[1] She noted asymmetrical power dynamics are often present in such partnerships, as health systems typically have more money and resources than partnering organizations, and they are often the largest employers in their communities. Practices to mitigate the asymmetrical power dynamics between a community and collaborating health system can strengthen partnerships.

Partnering to Address Health Disparities in Memphis, Tennessee

Egregious race-related health disparities in terms of diabetes, cancer, suicide and homicide, and infant health are at play in Memphis, Tennessee, said Cutts. The city's cardiovascular disease mortality rate in 2010 for African Americans was twice that of white people. In 2010, the average white family's income was approximately double that of the African American family. In 2006, the Methodist Le Bonheur Healthcare (MLH) system formed a partnership with more than 700 religious congregations—86 percent of which were African American organizations. Led by Reverend Bobby Baker, director of faith and community partnerships at MLH, and Gary Gunderson, vice president for faith and health at Wake

---

[1] More information about the Congregational Health Network is available at https://www.methodisthealth.org/about-us/faith-and-health/congregational-health-network (accessed March 19, 2021).

Forest Baptist Medical Center, CHN was created to improve access and health status for the entire community. The network's efforts are referred to as the Memphis Model.

Cutts stated that CHN's robust commitment to improved community health is evident in its outcomes (Barnes et al., 2014; Cutts, 2011; Thompson et al., 2018). During the first 25 months of the initiative, medical charges for the CHN patient population were $4 million less in aggregate than for the control group, which was matched for age, sex, and diagnosis related group. The mortality rate was decreased by half for CHN patients. Across the All Patient Refined Diagnosis Related Groups, the period until hospital readmission was 69 days longer for CHN patients. Cutts noted that in spite of distrust in the community, significantly more CHN members navigated to hospice and home health services. The efforts of Wellness Without Walls, a targeted, place-based population health initiative, yielded an 8.9 percent decrease in charity care in one of the poorest zip codes in the country, 38109.

Lessons from the Aligning Forces for Quality Grant

In 2009, MLH received an Aligning Forces for Quality grant from the Robert Wood Johnson Foundation. The health care system launched an effort to standardize racial, ethnic, and language preferences for data collection. The process began with data collection across the hospitals in the MLH system, an activity that had not been performed prior to this effort. In response to patient feedback, MLH added a biracial/multiracial option. Another arm of the study examined ideal measures of cardiac care through racial, ethnic, and language lenses. Cutts stated that Methodist North Hospital, an MLH facility, surpassed ideal measures of cardiac care goals at rates of 96 percent for patients with congestive heart failure and at 100 percent for those with acute myocardial infarction (AMI) who were admitted to the hospital. This level of care was delivered regardless of race, ethnicity, or language, said Cutts. However, a grim disparity emerged from additional data. African Americans inside or in route to the emergency department were dying of sudden cardiac death at twice the rate of their white counterparts. Additionally, readmissions were lower for African Americans than for white patients. Furthermore, in examining the age of the prehospital sudden cardiac deaths, a disparity surfaced with the mean age for African American deaths at 58 years compared to 66.5 years for whites.

Cutts said these findings represented a disconnection between the values, metrics, and leaders of the health system and those of the community. While hospital leadership was pleased with ideal measures of cardiac care goals being surpassed at high rates, CHN members and leaders were horrified at the rate at which African Americans in their community were dying, and they demanded action of the health system, said Cutts. This disconnection highlighted an important lessons: to achieve community health equity, the work must be community led and initiated. Additionally, health systems can become teachable through longstanding, humble relationships with the community. Cutts noted that Gary Shorb, chief executive officer of MLH at that time, allowed transparent sharing of this disparity data with the media. In spite of some pushback from some partners, Shorb maintained that community input was necessary in moving the needle on this health disparity.

Addressing Racial Cardiac Disparities

A series of internal MLH meetings focused on dialogues around race disparities, explicitly discussing topics that previously were not spoken about. The CHN liaison council, a self-organized group of women, allowed MLH access to a broader group of 75 CHN liaisons to share data and receive input on why African Americans were dying at higher rates in route to or inside of the emergency department. This community intelligence revealed that distrust of hospitals is common among African Americans. Cutts referenced the book *Medical Apartheid: The Dark History of Medical Experimentation on Black Americans from Colonial Times to the Present*, which outlines the source of this distrust (Washington, 2006). Furthermore, lack of health insurance was a barrier to accessing care for many people in the community. Medical fatalism—a hopelessness regarding future health status—was also expressed as a contributing factor.

During an interactive, educational session with community members, CHN shared information about the effect of race on best practice in medication treatment. Research trials are conducted with a majority of white populations, typically beginning with white males and then extending to white females, said Cutts. Only in recent decades have racial and ethnic differences been explored through studies with additional subgroups. During the session, medical professionals shared that calcium channel blockers tend to be more effective than beta blockers in preventing future heart attacks in African Americans. Community members discussed that heart medication side effects, such as erectile dysfunction, affect compliance in taking medication. Cutts recalled that when CHN explained that prodromal and presenting symptoms for AMI differ by race, and that a major symptom for African American and Hispanic women is debilitating fatigue, a collective gasp was heard in the room. Community members shared that many underresourced women work multiple jobs while simultaneously providing care to family members, making fatigue common. The CHN staff members advised the group to encourage any female friends or relatives experiencing fatigue to get prompt medical attention.

The MLH Quality Team shared information with medical staff about best-practice medications for minoritized populations. In collaboration with the community, CHN developed culturally sensitive, low literacy teach back tools on preventing heart failure and AMI to be given to patients during hospital discharge. Other discharge materials were decreased to draw patient attention to the most important health information, bringing the total number of discharge papers from 48 pages to only a few pieces of paper. The CHN Academy co-branded with MLH and incorporated the teach back tools into chronic disease and community health workforce courses. This effort was designed to familiarize people in the community with the acute symptoms that necessitate an immediate trip to the hospital.

Effect and Implications of CHN Efforts

These collective efforts resulted in a 15 percent decrease in the disparity for sudden cardiac death for African Americans from 2010 to 2012. Given the importance of language, Cutts noted that the Systems Bioethics Committee changed its name to the Ethics and Equity Committee. Sunny Anand, an intensivist at MLH Le Bonheur Children's Hospital, began looking at Hispanic data and discovered that Hispanic children were dying in the neonatal intensive care unit and the pediatric intensive care unit at almost four times the rate of African American and white children (Anand et al., 2015). Anand initiated a 3-year, multilevel community and hospital intervention that decreased this disparity.

Social complexity means that life exists within an interconnected web of systems and relationships that shape social and physical contexts, said Cutts. Like community power, social complexity is difficult to measure, and traditional tools and metrics are inadequate to do so, which calls for creativity and mixed-methods approaches. Additionally, iterative learning cycles and formative evaluation—such as plan-do-study-act cycles—allow metrics to be used expeditiously to refine processes, programs, and policy. Furthermore, measurement must be non-extractive, Cutts maintained. Data belong to the community and should be created, built, measured, analyzed, and continually interpreted with the community. Finally, building trust and integrity within a program are more important than the rigor of the design or metrics. Cutts concluded by emphasizing that "a healthy community is a powerful community."

COMMUNITY EMPOWERMENT AND HEALTH EQUITY: PRACTICING COMMUNITY-BASED PARTICIPATORY RESEARCH IN THE TIME OF COVID-19

Parajón stated that as both a physician and a public health practitioner, her training in these two areas has taught her to see patients as individuals and to see communities. She uses community-based participatory research (CBPR) maps to visualize the work toward equity. CBPR is "a collaborative effort between multisector stakeholders who gather and use research and data to build on the strengths and priorities of the community and use multilevel strategies to improve health and social equity" (Wallerstein et al., 2017). This definition drives the CBPR conceptual model,[2] which visualizes connections between four areas: (1) the context of a health outcome; (2) partnership processes; (3) intervention programs, research, and evaluation; and (4) health and social justice outcomes. The model explores factors of each of these areas and the influence the areas have upon one another.[3] Parajón noted that this model is based on Paulo Freire's work, which defined empowerment as "a dialogue process in which passive subjects become participatory actors" (Freire, 1970). She explained CBPR is a plan-do-study-act model that can involve a time investment in building trust. However, once that trust has been created between an organization and community members, the model can using a rapid cycle of listening, dialoguing, and taking action within a community. During the COVID-19 pandemic, using a rapid cycle approach has been helpful in developing effective, time-sensitive services, said Parajón.

Practical Application of Community-Based Participatory Research

Until recently, Parajón served as a physician in a large congregant shelter for people experiencing homelessness. Located outside of Albuquerque, New Mexico, the Heading Home shelter buses residents daily for the 30-minute drive to and from the city.[4] The COVID-19 pandemic created high-risk situations both in the bus rides and within the congregant setting, where many residents are housed together in the dormitory. Parajón noted that the shelter also has a number of asylum seekers, and this presents additional challenges to address. A multisector, community

---

[2] More information about the community-based participatory research model is available at https://cpr.unm.edu/research-projects/cbpr-project/cbpr-model.html (accessed April 15, 2021).

[3] More information about this model and additional CBPR tools is available at https://engageforequity.org (accessed March 20, 2021).

[4] More information about Heading Home is available at https://headinghome.org (accessed March 20, 2021).

coalition–based partnership came together to provide COVID-19 prevention and response efforts for people experiencing homelessness. Dubbing themselves the "Corona Crushers," the coalition included city and state departments, universities, Medical Reserve Corps, outreach medicine providers, community health workers, and Heading Home shelter staff.

Outcome Identification

Using the CBPR methodologies, the coalition began by identifying outcomes for health equity by speaking with people experiencing homelessness. This community was disproportionately affected by the COVID-19 virus, with many community members expressing fear about feeling unable to keep themselves safe. The overarching health equity outcome identified was reducing the spread of COVID-19 for people experiencing homelessness who do not have homes where they can self-isolate. Parajón outlined desired long-term outcomes, including positive community transformation, improved health by way of decreased COVID-19 infections, and increased access to COVID-19 immunizations. Additionally, desired intermediate outcomes were identified, including power sharing within the multisector coalition and the community, developing a sustained partnership, enacting policy change in universities and in the community to help them find their power, and facilitating individual and agency capacity.

Context of the Health Issue

The coalition then looked at the context of COVID-19 risk for people experiencing homelessness (Kaplan, 2020). Parajón explained that context within the CBPR model involves the following areas: health issue importance, social and structural, political and policy, capacity and readiness, and collaboration trust and mistrust. In this case, the important health issue was the higher rates of illness and comorbidity in the homeless population in comparison to the general population. Social and structural inequities involved the inability to self-isolate within the congregate nature of living in the shelter. The policy and politics contextual aspects included support from a number of departments and agencies. Capacity and readiness involved the capacity of the numerous partners involved in the coalition. The history of trust and collaboration pertained to the year of bimonthly meetings that had taken place.

Partnership Processes

Parajón emphasized the importance of various aspects of partnerships, including who the partners are, how they relate to one another, and how the partnership is structured. She stated that partnerships that have deliberate communication, integrate community knowledge, and foster trust tend to have better outcomes. Structures that facilitate power-building practices are also helpful, said Parajón. She noted a partnership practices guide that involves surveys that partnering organizations complete together to identify practices that need to change or be improved upon. Additionally, a partnership data report is generated that highlights indicators shown to improve outcomes, such as the percentage of the budget that is allocated for community spending, final approval, and control of resources.

Program Processes

The Corona Crushers coalition focused on actions that could be completed by communities, eliminating the need to rely on universities, said Parajón. The partners listened to one another, coordinated on a daily basis with partnering organizations and with a medical team of health care providers, and co-developed medical pathways, a volunteer call system, medical coverage, testing sites, and isolation pods. Furthermore, the coalition fostered trust, built community, and facilitated equity and power. As COVID-19 can spread quickly in a shelter, it was important that agencies had clear roles and responsibilities and subscribed to specific organizational practices. Parajón noted that how things are done is as important as what is done. Working alongside shelter staff and community health workers, the coalition established empowering practices to build capacity and integrate local knowledge. COVID-19 screening and testing, isolation, social distancing, early medical care, and partnerships were key elements of the response.

Quarantine areas were developed in collaboration with the community of people experiencing homelessness. In creating quarantine pods, a feedback co-learning process was used in which data from homeless shelter residents was incorporated into the program design. This extended to improving food quality and treating people with kindness. Parajón remarked that after feedback was received that people in quarantine were not being treated nicely, intervention to emphasize the importance of kindness resulted in improved behavior. She noted that helping people quarantine effectively helps slow the spread of COVID-19. Pandemic funding was used for wellness hotel stays that served multiple purposes: the short-term need for isolation and the long-term need for transitional housing. The community expressed confusion about who needed to wear specific types of masks or take other precautions, so the coalition's medical students and undergrads developed visual guides that were easy to understand.

Power Dynamics in Community-Based Participatory Research

Parajón stated that aspects of power building to focus on in measuring impact include emancipatory power, deliberative communication in partnering practices, valuing community knowledge and co-learning processes, and social justice and equity outcomes (Wallerstein et al., 2019). She outlined some specific effects of the coalition's efforts. The first was the ability to quickly react to a large COVID-19 outbreak that took place in October 2020 and comprised the majority of New Mexico's positivity rate that day. The team regrouped and successfully advocated for rapid testing equipment from the Department of Health. As a team and as a community, they reduced COVID-19 infections at the shelter to a rate lower than the community rate. Parajón reported that the risk of COVID-19 infection was currently lower in the shelter than out in the community. The second effect was an alignment of efforts through CBPR and community leadership that involved shared outcomes and collaboration in examining context and developing programs. Third, a new protocol was developed that can now be used in other shelters, congregant settings, and with asylum seekers. Fourth, the coalition worked to build capacity in the students and shelter residents and in resources such as sheltering-in-place beds and supplies. The CBPR pathway—analyzing contexts together, partnering in ways that improve programs, and the resulting social equity outcomes—guides participants in using data through each of these steps. Parajón remarked that CBPR is about "showing up, being who you are, listening intently, believing in social justice, and taking action for social change."

DISCUSSION

Context and Relational Aspects of Power Building

Yu noted Speer's emphasis on the role of community dynamics in driving strategic decisions, prioritizing the measuring of community powers, focusing on relational qualities of power building and community change, and examining longitudinal multilevel relationships. She asked the panelists to speak to the connections between one another's presentations. Speer highlighted the nuance, complexity, and sophisticated practice taking place within community power building. This involves truly listening to people and thinking relationally. Investment by researchers in the deeper methods discussed will enable greater understanding of how power is developed and manifested, said Speer. Yu added that several panelists spoke about context around a health issue, and that this is a challenging component for evaluators and researchers to capture.

Parajón stated that she has worked with the CBPR model in New Mexico and in Nicaragua, and she has found that having a guide and checklists for partners to use facilitates implementation of the model. A checklist is used for each area of the CBPR model: context, partnership, program, and outcome. These include assessing whether staff have cultural humility and whether they are engaging in various partnering practices. Expanding beyond the actual intervention, the list of partnering practices for people to learn and use focuses attention on how staff are interacting with people and building and supporting relationships. She noted that just as memorandums of understanding are used to outline how money and resources will be allocated, checklists for the CBPR components frame how people will relate to one another throughout the processes.

Wright remarked that a contextual aspect of studying community building—which both fascinates and frustrates him—is that community work has been taking place for many years. A current study of community-building work, or a recent initiative like BHC, can give the appearance that this type of work is new. However, an important element of context for researchers in this field to understand is that they are measuring a continuum of work that has been ongoing in communities for a long time, he emphasized. In contrast to a discrete effort that is initiated and results in change that can be measured, power-building initiatives may have amplification effects, but researchers are not creating new work. This is a challenge to address in determining how to study power-building efforts, said Wright.

Cutts added that in her work with CHN in Memphis, she was as an embedded researcher on a medical team integrated into the community group. She attended all community events from the beginning of the initiative, and she helped develop celebratory services and worship events. Cutts noted that congregational leaders emphasized the value of relationships, encouraging team members to "be there for the long run, not just for photo ops." She said this relational component builds trust and is critical to evaluation efforts. Wright remarked that in the absence of the embedded evaluator role that Cutts described, evaluation can resemble archaeology—that is, a process of piecing together information from an outside perspective. He added that even BHC's work can sometimes be prone to that dynamic. This type of reconstruction often leads to transactional issues or an incomplete picture of what took place, but this can be avoided by evaluators embedding themselves in the community from the beginning, said Wright.

The Evolving Nature of Theory in Power Building

Yu commented on being open to evolving theories of change, noting that BHC did not develop its theory of change until 2013, and that indicators centering power as an end in itself, and not just a means, were not added until 2017. As a foundation, TCE uses an adaptive learning mode that is responsive to community, she added. Yu asked panelists to comment on the process of evaluating interventions or outcomes without being wedded to a specific framework or theory. Martinez stated that this process can be frustrating for consultants and evaluators. Power building is not one distinct intervention with a well-defined program model featuring a beginning and end that can be assessed for fidelity. Rather, it is a process of constant improvement. Realizing that this work around power building, resistance, and survival has been taking place for centuries can be helpful in shifting to that perspective, she noted. While the absence of a linear theory of change and measures can be challenging, it is also powerful to wade into the complexity of the dynamics, striving to improve the ability to capture what is taking place, said Martinez.

Noting the flexibility needed in addressing power in all its various forms, Parajón stated that she appreciates that the CBPR model involves a dialectic process in simultaneously serving as a tool for planning, evaluation, and reflection. With this model, everyone—medical practitioners and people experiencing homelessness alike—learns together through the practice of listening, dialogue, and taking action. The power of this approach was apparent in the COVID-19 environment, in which situations and information evolved rapidly, said Parajón. The people living and working together in the shelter continually used a reflective cycle, and the collaborative act of using this cycle built trust. She added how important collaboration is in defining the community's priorities, as this leads to clear outcomes that everyone collectively works toward.

Transparency and Confidentiality in Community Data

A participant asked how to approach long-term data efforts that protect communities of color, given that this data can be used by those who oppose your efforts. Yu noted that BHC is giving care to protecting confidentiality in a survey currently being developed. Wright responded that BHC evaluation work involves a large ecosystem of individuals and organizations. To support, build, and weave that network together, BHC surveys community organizations and partners. They discuss the importance of transparency and creating a shared community asset. However, he noted there are risks with transparency, as the data they are collecting could be valuable to someone with ill intentions toward the outcomes

BHC's network strives to achieve. Therefore, BHC tries to anticipate potential unintended consequences in determining whether or not to make data available. Wright said this raises the issue of responsibility in creating a learning system, as the consequences of learning engines can be positive in building power but there is potential for destructive ramifications. Yu said it is critical to develop systems that serve power builders' strategy capacity but do not tip off the opposition.

Remote Community Engagement

A participant in a modified remote CBPR approach for a place-based intervention asked how to engage with the community without being physically present. Parajón replied that video conferencing is an option if community members have Internet access. In the shelter, residents did not have phones, and physical presence was required. However, when lack of Internet access is not a barrier, video conferencing platforms such as Zoom make remote community-building activities that build trust possible. She has worked on projects using CBPR with health councils via Zoom, and this platform enables progress in the absence of in-person interactions. Additionally, she uses Jamboard, an interactive digital whiteboard, that works well for CBPR model planning and visioning. Yu added that geography and time constraints can make it difficult to be in the community, yet relationship and trust building require it. She said COVID-19 is forcing people to interface in a different way, via video conferencing, and that this requires access issues to be addressed.

Community-Building Learning Engine

A participant asked for additional information about BHC's emerging platform for open source, collective action learning, such as its design features, important elements of infrastructure, and timeline. Wright replied that rather than creating an evaluation, BHC is working to develop a connected analytic engine and data ecosystem. The concept involves an extensive catalog of practices and their connections to one another. Eventually, TCE will invite partners to this catalog. The universal coding and connecting system developed by BHC will potentially enable a user with a specific question of interest to easily sort through data elements along applicable dimensions. The confidentiality concerns previously discussed come into play in determining a process for extracting information from the data ecosystem, said Wright. He remarked that the goal is to have a repository that thinkers and researchers working to advance the field can take advantage of. Local control in numerous communities has played a strong role in the evolution of BHC, leading it to become a laboratory for innovation. Wright remarked there is much to learn from all that activity, and it is hoped the learning engine will enable lots of minds to come together to learn as much as possible from the data.

Power-Building Efforts in Memphis, Tennessee

A participant interested in the Memphis Model asked about the extent to which power-building efforts have continued in Memphis and about any challenges preventing a wider diffusion of the model. Cutts stated that she now lives in North Carolina, but she is aware that some community-building efforts in Memphis are ongoing. She said CHN has entered a latent period owing to leadership changes, which could send a negative signal to the community regarding community power. However, faith community partnerships have endured for hundreds of years, and will continue to do so in spite of pandemics and leadership changes, she remarked. Leaders approach power differently. Some leaders are open to creating space for horizontal power differentials in which the community's power, intelligence, agency, and capacity are valued, while other leaders are not invested in that view. Cutts stated that the leaders involved in the Memphis Model intentionally held space open for community members to occupy, but she is unclear as to whether that continues to be the case. Leadership within health systems and within the community greatly affect how power is manifested. She added that the 2007 infant mortality rate for African American babies in Memphis was the same as the rate in Zimbabwe, and that this has since improved.

Summarizing Reflections

Ray Baxter, trustee of Blue Shield of California Foundation, shared several reflections about the workshop:

- Social determinants drive health but power defines, drives, and shapes those social determinants. The field of community health improvement needs to move from a technocratic approach toward a more democratic approach to health that values people above all.
- Narratives from communities are more than an additional source of evidence, more than another tool, not just one more input into decisions. They help us confront the dominant narratives that serve power and that have already shaped what questions are even considered. Those dominant narratives can normalize racism, white supremacy, misogyny, selfish individualism, and economic exploitation.

- There is already a body of knowledge, expertise, and proven practices around community power building. There is a diverse array of practitioners and organizations devoted to doing this and supporting it, and people working in the health field need to connect more fully with it.
- Relationships are just as important as technical solutions, not just institutional relationships but personal, economic, and cross-cultural relationships.
- Investing in leaders, particularly positioning youth and residents to lead in their communities and in our institutions is critical.

Baxter's final observation was that at the present moment, some institutions are failing communities and that "this is a time when transformational change is possible."

A

References

Achor, S., A. Reece, G. R. Kellerman, and A. Robichaux. 2018. 9 out of 10 people are willing to earn less money to do more-meaningful work. *Harvard Business Review*, November 6.

Anand, K. J., R. J. Sepanski, K. Giles, S. H. Shah, and P. D. Juarez. 2015. Pediatric intensive care unit mortality among Latino children before and after a multilevel health care delivery intervention. *JAMA Pediatrics* 169(4):383–390.

Ball, S., and G. A. Bogatz. 1970. *The first year of Sesame Street: An evaluation.* Princeton, NJ: Educational Testing Service.

Barnes, P., T. Cutts, S. Dickinson, H. Guo, D. Squires, S. Bowman, and G. Gunderson. 2014. Methods for managing and analyzing electronic medical records: A formative examination of a hospital-congregation-based intervention. *Population Health Management* 17(5):279–286.

Caring Across Generations. 2020. *The importance of building narrative and cultural power: A culture change primer.* New York: Caring Across Generations.

City of Long Beach Department of Health and Human Services. 2013. *Community health assessment.* Long Beach, CA: City of Long Beach.

Cutler, J. J., G. S. Parker, S. Rosen, B. Prenney, R. Healey, and G. G. Caldwell. 1986. Childhood leukemia in Woburn, Massachusetts. *Public Health Reports (Washington, D.C.: 1974)* 101(2):201–205.

Cutts, T. 2011. The Memphis Congregational Health Network Model: Grounding ARHAP theory. In *When religion and health align.* Pietermaritzburg, South Africa: Cluster Publications. Pp. 193–209.

Epstein, R., J. Blake, and T. González. 2017. *Girlhood interrupted: The erasure of black girls' childhood.* Washington, DC: Georgetown Law Center on Poverty and Inequality.

Freire, P. 1970. *Pedagogy of the oppressed.* New York: Herder and Herder.

Gunderson, G., and L. Pray. 2009. *Five fundamentals to change the way you live your life.* Nashville, TN: Abingdon Press.

Han, H. 2020. *Reflections on measuring community power.* The Johns Hopkins University. https://static1.squarespace.com/static/5ee2c6c3c085f746bd33f80e/t/5f8f0e14736c6833fda80f7a/1603210772405/20201020.MeasuringPower.pdf (accessed February 21, 2021).

Healy, R., and S. Hinson. 2005. Movement strategy for organizers. In *Rhyming Hope and History: Activists, Academics and Social Movement Scholarship*, edited by D. Croteau, W. Hoynes, and C. Ryan. Minneapolis, MN: University of Minnesota Press.

Healy, R. 2018. *The three faces of power*. Grassroots Power Project. https://grassrootspolicy.org/wp-content/uploads/2018/05/GPP_34FacesOfPower.pdf (accessed August 20, 2021).

Hogan, A., and B. Roberts. 2015. Occupational employment projections to 2024. *Monthly Labor Review*, December.

Human Impact Partners and Right to the City Alliance. 2020. *A primer on power, housing justice, and health equity*. Oakland, CA: Human Impact Partners and Right to the City Alliance.

Ito, J., and M. Pastor. 2018. *A pivot to power: Lessons from the California Endowment's building healthy communities about place, health, and philanthropy*. Los Angeles, CA: USC Dornsife Program for Environmental and Regional Equity.

Kaplan, E. 2020. Exposed and at risk. *Albuquerque Journal*, March 15. https://www.abqjournal.com/1432018/exposed-and-atrisk.html (accessed March 20, 2021).

King, M. L., Jr., 1967. *Beyond Vietnam*. Stanford University, The Martin Luther King, Jr. Research and Education Institute. https://kinginstitute.stanford.edu/king-papers/documents/beyond-vietnam (accessed March 1, 2021).

Miller, C. C., S. Goldmacher, and T. Kaplan. 2020. Biden announces $775 billion plan to help working parents and caregivers. *The New York Times*, August 26.

Ortega y Gasset, J. 1914. *Meditaciones del Quijote*. Madrid, Spain: Residencia de Estudiantes.

Pascal, R., M. Sternin, and J. Sternin. 2010. *The power of positive deviance*. Boston, MA: Harvard Business Press.

Pastor, M., J. Ito, and W. M. 2020. *Leading locally: A community power-building approach to structural change*. Los Angeles, CA: USC Equity Research Institute.

Poo, A.-j. 2019. The people who look after your children deserve basic rights. *The New York Times*, July 14.

Poo, A.-j., and B. W. Veghte. 2019. The big, feminist policy idea America's families have been waiting for. *The New York Times*, June 23.

Singhal, A. 2010. Communicating what works! Applying the positive deviance approach in health communication. *Health Communication* 25(6):605–606.

Singhal, A. In press. *The art of positive deviance: A radically different way of solving the world's toughest problems*. New Delhi, India: The Change Designers Press.

Singhal, A., and L. Dura. 2009. *Protecting children from exploitation and trafficking: Using the Positive Deviance approach in Uganda and Indonesia*. Washington, DC: Save the Children.

Singhal, A., and P. J. Svenkerud. 2018. Diffusion of evidence-based interventions or practice-based positive deviations. *Journal of Development Communication* 29(2):54–64.

Singhal, A., and P. J. Svenkerud. 2019. Flipping the diffusion of innovations paradigm: Embracing the positive deviance approach to social change. *Asia Pacific Media Educator*. July 1–13. doi: 10.1177/1326365X19857010.

Singhal, A., P. Buscell, and C. Lindberg. 2010. *Inviting everyone: Healing healthcare through positive deviance*. Bordentown, NJ: Plexus Press

Speer, P., J. Gupta, and K. Haapenen. 2020. *A research agenda for developing and measuring community power for health equity*. Nashville, TN: Vanderbilt University.

Sternin, J., and R. Choo. 2000. The power of positive deviancy. An effort to reduce malnutrition in Vietnam offers an important lesson about managing change. *Harvard Business Review* 78(1):14–15.

Thompson, M. P., P. S. B. Podila, C. Clay, J. Sharp, S. Bailey-DeLeeuw, A. J. Berkley, B. G. Baker, and T. M. Waters. 2018. Community navigators reduce hospital utilization in super-utilizers. *American Journal of Managed Care* 24(2):70–76.

University of Wisconsin Population Health Institute. 2011. *County health rankings state report 2011: California*. Madison, WI: University of Wisconsin Population Health Institute.

University of Wisconsin Population Health Institute. 2020. *County health rankings state report 2020: California*. Madison, WI: University of Wisconsin Population Health Institute.

USC (University of Southern California) Dornsife Equity Research Institute. 2020. *A primer on community power, place, and structural change*. Los Angeles, CA: USC Dornslife Equity Research Institute.

USC PERE (Program for Environmental and Regional Equity). 2018. *California health and justice for all power-building landscape: A preliminary assessment*. Los Angeles, CA: USC Dornsife Program for Environmental and Regional Equity.

Wallerstein, N., B. Duran, J. G. Oetzel, and M. Minkler. 2017. *Community-based participatory research for health: Advancing social and health equity*. Hoboken, NJ: Jossey-Bass.

Wallerstein, N., M. Muhammad, S. Sanchez-Youngman, P. Rodriguez Espinosa, M. Avila, E. A. Baker, S. Barnett, L. Belone, M. Golub, J. Lucero, I. Mahdi, E. Noyes, T. Nguyen, Y. Roubideaux, R. Sigo, and B. Duran. 2019. Power dynamics in community-based participatory research: A multiple-case study analysis of partnering contexts, histories, and practices. *Health Education & Behavior* 46(Suppl 1):19S–32S.

Washington, H. A. 2006. *Medical apartheid: The dark history of medical experimentation on black Americans from colonial times to the present*. New York: Doubleday Books.

B

Biosketches of Speakers, Moderators, and Planning Committee Members[1]

Ella Auchincloss, M.T.S., is The Rippel Foundation's director of enterprise innovation and a key contributor to Rippel's ReThink Health initiative's Hospital Systems in Transition and Portfolio Design for Healthier Regions projects. Auchincloss has spearheaded many resident engagement efforts for Rippel's ReThink Health initiative, coaching a wide variety of partner organizations and teams in change leadership and developing Community Activation for System Stewardship, in which she and her team advised the Centers for Medicare & Medicaid Service's Quality Improvement Organization Leadership, Organizing in Action program. She also directed a research project exploring tax credits' potential as a source of sustainable financing for population health.

Before joining Rippel, Auchincloss founded the Leadership Development Initiative, a faith-based teaching and coaching program for resident outreach. In 2015, she was awarded the Barbara C. Harris Award for Social Justice by the Episcopal City Mission in Boston, Massachusetts, for her founding of the Leadership Development Initiative. She is also a fellow of the Leading Change Network at Harvard University's Kennedy School of Government. Prior to her work in resident engagement, Auchincloss worked in the financial services sector. Auchincloss received an M.T.S. from the Harvard Divinity School and a B.S. from Babson College.

---

[1] * denotes planning committee member; † denotes roundtable member.

LaTosha Brown is an organizer, philanthropic consultant, activist, singer/songwriter, and co-founder of the Black Voters Matter Fund, a power-building, Southern-based civic engagement organization, and the Black Voters Matter Capacity Building Institute. She is the principal owner of TruthSpeaks Consulting, LLC, a philanthropy advisory consulting firm in Atlanta, Georgia, and the project director of Grantmakers for Southern Progress. She also works to eliminate human suffering through her vision of the Southern Black Girls & Women's Consortium. As a catalyst for change and social strategist, her national and global efforts have been known to organize, inspire, and catapult people into action—enabling them to build power and wealth for themselves and their community. She is most known for her philanthropic efforts as an effective fundraiser and resource person having raised millions of dollars to support social justice causes and created projects that bring more investments into marginalized communities. Brown's global thoughts toward people, ideas, and money have opened doors for her to maximize her voice in the United States and more than 30 countries abroad. She is currently leading several international efforts to provide training, support, and funding for women-led institutions based in Guyana, Senegal, Belize, and Tanzania.

Brown works to shift the narrative of African Americans through media, campaigns, and nonprofit projects. Featured on CNN, HBO, MSNBC, and Fox, among others, she also proudly serves as the founder of Saving OurSelves Coalition, a community-led disaster relief organization that helped hundreds of families in the aftermath of Hurricane Katrina. Currently, she serves on the board of the National Coalition on Black Civic Participation, the Southern Documentary Fund, the U.S. Human Rights Network, and the Congressional Progressive Caucus Center. Brown has received a number of awards, including the 2010 White House Champion of Change Award, the 2006 Spirit of Democracy Award, the Louis Burnham Award for Human Rights, and the Liberty Bell Award. Brown received a B.A. in political science and government from Auburn University at Montgomery in Alabama.

Michelle Carrillo is the director of programs and community solutions at the Humboldt Area Foundation (HAF), a community foundation working to promote and encourage generosity, leadership, and inclusion in a four-county rural region in northern California and the southern Oregon coast. In Carrillo's new role, she is part of a team dedicated to tackling long-term systemic change to foster a thriving, just, healthy, and equitable region. Prior to this new leadership role, Carrillo served as the director for Del Norte and Tribal Land's Building Healthy Communities Initiative, a 10-year, place-based health initiative funded by The California Endowment and housed at the Wild Rivers Community Foundation (WRCF), an affiliate of HAF. In 2019, the Robert Wood Johnson Foundation recognized Del Norte County as one of the 12 finalists for the nation's Culture of Health Prize.

Carrillo joined HAF/WRCF in 2015 after graduating from Southern Oregon University and working for 5 years at the Oregon State University School of Public Health through the Extension Service. The first grant Carrillo ever wrote was to HAF/WRCF, which enabled her to co-found an award winning 4-H Surfing and Outdoor Stewardship Program at the age of 22. Carrillo's role in large-scale regional health equity initiatives has allowed her to work alongside young leaders, community members, sovereign nations, and system leaders tackling intractable systemic problems, applying empathy research, social innovation, and entrepreneurial thinking in the field. She has supported a variety of community-led projects using the human-centered design and systems transformation for equity approach to address a broad set of issues ranging from children's literacy to the health of the nonprofit sector.

Teresa Cutts, Ph.D., is the research assistant professor at the Wake Forest School of Medicine's (WFSOM's) Public Health Sciences Division, where she serves as a researcher, program developer, and more for the FaithHealth Division. She also holds appointments in the Maya Angelou Center for Health Equity. Since 2017, she has served as the principal investigator (PI) for the Empowerment Project's homeless outreach and case management at WFSOM. Prior to her time at WFSOM, Cutts served as the director of research for innovation at Methodist Le Bonheur Healthcare's Interfaith Health Program Center of Excellence in Faith and Health. She worked explicitly in the area of evaluation and program development for Methodist's Memphis Model Congregational Health Network, Religious Health Assets mapping, and Integrated Health for congregations, community, and clergy. She is the academic liaison to the Stakeholder Health learning collaborative. Cutts has also served as the PI or the co-PI on dozens of grants, including those funded by the Robert Wood Johnson Foundation, the Centers for Disease Control and Prevention, the Komen Foundation, and the Avon Foundation, working often on projects to improve health equity and the lives of the underserved and most vulnerable.

From 2001 to 2005, Cutts was the director of program development at the Church Health Center, a comprehensive, faith-based health program for the underserved. She held a joint clinical appointment in preventive medicine and psychiatry at The University of Texas at Austin, the University of Memphis School of Public Health, and still holds an appointment at the Memphis Theological Seminary. She is a visiting professor at the University of Cape Town School of Family Medicine and Public Health and has co-authored or published numerous book chapters and articles. She was the co-editor and helped co-author many chapters in the book *Stakeholder Health: Insights from New Systems of Health*. Cutts has also worked as a staff psychologist at Baptist Memorial Hospital, as a private practitioner at the Memphis Center for Women and Families, and she served as a consultant to the National Institutes of Health gastroparesis multisite consortium. She completed her Ph.D. and M.A. at the University of Mississippi.

Rashida Ferdinand, M.F.A., is the founder and the executive director of Sankofa. A fifth-generation homeowner and visual artist in the Lower 9th Ward of New Orleans, Louisiana, Ferdinand comes from a family of community health practitioners and social justice leaders. She founded Sankofa with a team of community stakeholders in 2008 to create a local environment that promotes positive health and environmental sustainability. Sankofa's food access programs focus on building a healthy food system in vulnerable communities of New Orleans. These efforts are designed to ensure resilience, community empowerment, and equity. Ferdinand completed her B.F.A. at Howard University and her M.F.A. at Syracuse University. She is a graduate of the fourth cohort of Goldman Sach's 10,000 Small Businesses program and currently represents Sankofa on the Xavier University LaCats New Orleans Community Advisory Board, the Louisiana State University and the Southern University Ag Center Orleans Parish Advisory Leadership Council, the Mid South Transdisciplinary Collaborative Center on Health Disparities, the Greater New Orleans Water Collaborative, and the New Orleans Food Policy Advisory Committee.

Julie Fernandes, J.D., is an associate director for institutional accountability and individual liberty at the Rockefeller Family Fund in New York. Prior to joining the Rockefeller Family Fund, she served as the Open Society Foundation's director for voting rights and democracy. She also worked as a deputy assistant attorney general in the civil rights division in the Obama administration and as the special assistant for domestic policy to President Clinton. In addition, Fernandes served as the senior counsel and the senior policy analyst at the Leadership Conference for Civil & Human Rights, one of the nation's leading civil rights organizations. She has testified before Congress on voting rights issues and has authored several research reports and magazine pieces primarily in the areas of voting rights and criminal justice reform. Regarding her education, Fernandes received both her J.D. and B.A. from the University of Chicago and clerked for the Honorable Diane P. Wood at the U.S. Court of Appeals for the Seventh Circuit.

Ethan Frey is a program officer of the Ford Foundation's Cities and States team. In this role, he works in collaboration with programs across the foundation to develop and implement tailored grantmaking strategies in six states—Texas, Florida, Louisiana, New York, Michigan, and Minnesota—where the foundation will focus its work to build the capacity of people-centered ecosystems seeking long-term, statewide change over the next 5 years. Frey joined the Ford Foundation in 2013 as a program associate on the Civic Engagement and Government team. During his tenure, he has worked primarily on the foundation's organizing, voting rights, census, and voter engagement programs. Previously, Frey served as a regional field director in Columbus, Ohio, for the 2012 presidential campaign and before that as a field organizer in Toledo during the 2008 general election campaign. He also worked to unionize low-wage workers in Miami, Florida, as an organizer for the international trade union Unite Here, which represents food service, hotel, and gaming employees. At Project Renewal, a nonprofit social service provider, he worked to protect public benefits for low-income New Yorkers as a non-attorney civil legal advocate. Frey is a 2010 graduate of Westminster College in New Wilmington, Pennsylvania.

Roxanne Carrillo Garza, M.S.W., is the senior director of Healthy Richmond, a 10-year initiative funded by The California Endowment. She currently works with resident leaders, community-based organizations, base builders, and systems leaders to develop collective policy advocacy strategies to improve health, safety, school and neighborhood environments, and economic development opportunities in California. Garza works for RCF Connects (formerly the Richmond Community Foundation), which partners with the community to inspire leadership and to share the vision for work in five areas: community growth, health, restoring neighborhoods, education, and public safety. Prior to joining Healthy Richmond in 2013, Garza was a public health program manager for Contra Costa Health Services where she worked on environmental justice, alcohol policy, neighborhood improvements, and violence prevention efforts across Contra Costa County. Garza was the allocations and planning director for the United Way of Greater Los Angeles, Service Planning Area 1, and the program manager for El Nido Family Services, a social service nonprofit agency providing counseling and family support services to disadvantaged communities in Los Angeles County. Garza received her bachelor's degree in political science from California State University, Northridge, and her M.S.W. from the University of California, Los Angeles.

Gary Gunderson, D.Min., D.Div., M.Div.,*† oversees spiritual care services for patients, families, and medical center staff at the Wake Forest Baptist Medical Center. In his position, Gunderson supervises six departments: CareNet Counseling, Chaplaincy and Clinical Ministries, FaithHealth Education, Community Engagement, the Center for Congregational Health, and FaithHealthNC. He also nurtures the relationship with more than 4,300 Baptist congregations throughout North Carolina and other large networks of patients' faith groups. A recognized expert in congregations and health, Gunderson has previously served as the senior vice president of the Faith and Health Division of Methodist Le Bonheur Healthcare in Memphis, Tennessee. In his 7 years there, he developed a new model of congregational health that became widely known as the Memphis Model. Gunderson became involved in public health through his work with former President Jimmy Carter in Atlanta when he directed the Interfaith Health Program at the Carter Center for a decade. The Interfaith Health Program moved from the Carter Center to the Rollins School of Public Health at Emory University, where Gunderson became a research assistant professor in international health. He also served as a visiting professor in family medicine and community health at the University of Cape Town, South Africa.

Gunderson has worked extensively with the White House Office of Faith-Based and Neighborhood Partnerships. He serves as the secretary for Stakeholder Health, a group of 39 health systems committed to more effective engagement with the poor in their communities. He brought the Leading Causes of Life Initiative to Wake Forest Baptist, an international and interdisciplinary group of fellows working to build an intellectual foundation beyond the purely medical paradigm. He was the lead author for a 2015 paper based on this work and published by the National Academy of Medicine, *The Health of Complex Human Populations*. In addition to his role in faith and health ministries, Gunderson holds faculty appointments at the Wake Forest School of Divinity and in public health sciences. A Wake Forest University alumnus, Gunderson holds an M.Div. from Emory University in Atlanta, a D.Min. from the Interdenominational Theological Center in Atlanta, and an honorary D.Div. from the Chicago Theological Seminary.

Hahrie Han, Ph.D., is the inaugural director of the Stavros Niarchos Foundation Agora Institute, a professor of political science, and the faculty director of the P3 Research Lab at Johns Hopkins University. Han specializes in the study of civic and political participation, collective action, and organizing. She focuses particularly on the role that civic associations play in mobilizing participation in politics and building power for social and political change. Prior to her position at the institute, she served as the Anton Vonk Professor of Political Science and Environmental Politics at the University of California, Santa Barbara. From 2005 to 2015, she was an associate professor of political science at Wellesley College and a Robert Wood Johnson Health Policy Scholar at Harvard University from 2009 to 2011.

Han's work on participation, movement building, civic associations, primary elections, and congressional polarization has been published in outlets including the *American Political Science Review, American Sociological Review, American Journal of Sociology, Perspectives on Politics, British Journal of Political Science,* and elsewhere. Her work was awarded the 2013 Outstanding Academic Publication on Membership Organizations Award by the Institute for Nonprofit Research, Education, and Engagement. Han has also been involved in numerous efforts to make academic work relevant to the world of practice, including participating in the Social Science Research Council Anxieties of Democracy Participation Working Group; co-chairing the Research Council of the PICO National Network; serving on the advisory board of organizations like research4impact, the Climate Advocacy Lab, the Citizens Climate Lobby, and the DEMOS Integrated Race and Class Narrative Project; serving as the co-chair of the Civic Engagement Working Group at the Scholars Strategy Network; co-founding and co-directing the Project on Public Leadership and Action at Wellesley College, and participating on the steering committee of the Gettysburg Project. Through her research, she partners with a wide range of civic and political organizations in the United States, Australia, New Zealand, the United Kingdom, and elsewhere. She also acted as the co-convenor of a Policy Advisory Committee for the 2008 Obama campaign and served as the chair of the Advisory Committee to the U.S. Election Assistance Commission agency review team on the Obama-Biden transition team. She received her Ph.D. in American politics from Stanford University and her B.A. in American history and literature from Harvard University in 1997.

Richard Healey, Ph.D., M.P.H., M.A., is the senior advisor to the Grassroots Policy Project (GPP), which he founded in 1994. GPP is focused on long-term strategies for transformative change, in particular on power, ideology, and movement infrastructure. He is also the chair of the board of the Commonwealth Foundation. Throughout the 1960s and 1970s, Healey was active in the civil rights and antiwar movements. From 1970 to 1982, he helped found and lead the New American Movement, a socialist-feminist organization that merged into the Democratic Socialists of America. Healey also became involved in community environmental health organizing. During the 1980s he was involved in disarmament and anti-intervention activities. He was the director of the Coalition for a New

Foreign and Military Policy and *Nuclear Times* magazine. He also served as the director of the Institute for Policy Studies. Healey received a B.A. in mathematics from Reed College, an M.A. and a Ph.D. in mathematics from the University of California, Los Angeles, and an M.P.H. from the Harvard T.H. Chan School of Public Health.

Jonathan Heller, Ph.D., recently joined the Population Health Institute at the University of Wisconsin as a senior health equity fellow. He is the co-founder and until 2020 was the co-director of Human Impact Partners (HIP), a national nonprofit organization focused on bringing the power of public health to campaigns and social movements for a just society. Under Heller's leadership for 14 years, HIP became a national public health leader focused on changing policies related to the social determinants of health by supporting community-organizing groups and campaigns with research and advocacy; conducting leadership development, capacity building, and political education with public health agencies; organizing the public health community; and supporting narrative change initiatives. HIP is credited for advancing a focus on equity and community power building within public health. Heller is also a co-founder and the past president of the Society of Practitioners of Health Impact Assessment and serves on the board of Community Change. He received his bachelor's degree from Harvard University and Ph.D. from the University of California, Berkeley, and he served in the Peace Corps in Papua New Guinea.

Mimi Ho is the executive director at Movement Strategy Center (MSC) in Oakland, California. At MSC, Ho has supported the alliance-building work of core partners including the Climate Justice Alliance, the HEAL (Health Environment, Agriculture Labor) Food Alliance, and the United Workers Congress. As part of MSC's Leadership Team, Ho helped launch the Transitions Initiative, MSC's multimovement initiative to bring movement leaders and emerging leaders together to build multisystems social change grounded in relationships and personal transformation.

Ho has served as a trainer and a consultant with racial justice and immigrant rights groups on community and electoral organizing strategy, grassroots leadership development, organizational development, and fundraising. Her clients have included the Western States Center and the Chinese Progressive Association in San Francisco. Ho was the statewide field director and the co-director of Californians for Justice (CFJ) during electoral fights against several racist ballot initiatives in the 1990s—attacks on affirmative action, bilingual education, youth, labor, and gay marriage. During the No on 209 (anti-affirmative action) campaign Ho oversaw fieldwork in 13 field offices and 1,350 precincts across California. She led CFJ in introducing public jobs legislation in the California legislature. Ho was a coordinator for national health care campaign work at the Northwest Federation of Community Organizations (now the Alliance for a Just Society and People's Action), and provided organizing, legislative, and communications training; campaign strategy consultation; and in-the-field capacity building for statewide affiliates in Washington, Oregon, Idaho, and Montana. Ho later worked with the Asian Pacific Environmental Network (APEN) where she directed campaigns to build green, affordable housing in Oakland, to organize electronic workers in China, and to keep Chevron from expanding to dirtier crude in Richmond, California. She helped grow APEN's cutting-edge Asian Pacific American electoral operation and supported APEN's shift into statewide climate policy and organizing work.

Tony Iton, M.D., J.D., M.P.H., is the senior vice president for Healthy Communities at The California Endowment. In 2009, he began to oversee the organization's 10-year, multimillion-dollar statewide commitment to advance policies and forge partnerships to build healthy communities and a healthy California. He is also a lecturer of health policy and management at the University of California (UC), Berkeley, School of Public Health, and serves on the board of directors of the Public Health Institute, the Public Health Trust, the Prevention Institute and Jobs for the Future. In the past, Iton has served as both the director and the county health officer for the Alameda County Public Health Department. In that role, he oversaw the creation of an innovative public health practice designed to eliminate health disparities by tackling the root causes of poor health that limit the quality of life and life span in many of California's low-income communities. He has worked as an HIV disability rights attorney at the Berkeley Community Law Center, a health care policy analyst with the Consumers Union West Coast Regional Office, and as a physician and an advocate for the homeless at the San Francisco Public Health Department. Iton's primary focus includes the health of disadvantaged populations and the contributions of race, class, wealth, education, geography, and employment to health status. In February 2010, he was recognized by the California Legislative Black Caucus with the Black History Month Legends Award; on the floor of the California State Assembly he was presented with a resolution memorializing his life's work and achievements. Iton completed his B.S. at McGill University in Montreal, his J.D. and M.P.H. at UC Berkely, and his M.D. at the Johns Hopkins University School of Medicine.

Taj James is the co-founder, former executive director, and current board member of Movement Strategy Center (MSC) in Oakland, California. As part of MSC's transitions incubator, James recently cofounded Full

Spectrum Capital Partners, housed in the Innovation Center of MSC. Since 2001, James and MSC have served as a consistent source of social change innovation and leadership. At MSC, he helped launch and support new alliances such as Strong Families and the Climate Justice Alignment. James has also played a key role in building new funding collaboratives and strategies to increase investment in grassroots organizing and alliance building. These initiatives include the California Fund for Youth Organizing, the Move to End Violence Initiative, the California Alliance for Boys and Men of Color, and Building Healthy Communities.

Before launching MSC, James served as the director of youth policy and development at Coleman Advocates for Children and Youth, where he organized youth and community members around issues facing children, youth, and families. James's network and leadership building experience began in his role as the Western regional field organizer for the Black Student Leadership Network, a project of the Children's Defense Fund. He served on the steering committee for the PAC to defeat Proposition 21, a California ballot initiative that would spend billions to incarcerate thousands of youth with adults. James has provided board leadership for many nonprofits and philanthropic institutions such the Praxis Project, Youth United for Community Action, the Funders' Collaborative on Youth Organizing, and the California Fund for Youth Organizing. A graduate of Stanford University, he was a recipient of a Next Generation Leadership fellowship from The Rockefeller Foundation.

Carmen Llanes Pulido is the executive director of Go Austin/Vamos Austin and a second-generation community organizer working with neighborhoods and organizations in Austin's Eastern Crescent for the past 15 years. After receiving an interdisciplinary B.A. at the University of Chicago in environmental studies with a focus on the North American Free Trade Agreement and its effect on Mexican communities and international food systems, she returned to Austin to work at home as an environmental justice researcher and organizer for People Organized in Defense of Earth and her Resources in East Austin. She later ran a program at the nonprofit organization Marathon Kids called the Wellness Team Initiative, which engaged parents and teachers at 18 elementary schools in Austin's Eastern Crescent to increase fitness and nutrition opportunities in their communities. Llanes Pulido cares deeply about community relationships and intergenerational organizing and participates in public health, antiracist, and antidisplacement networks in Central Texas and across the country. She chaired the City of Austin's Hispanic/Latino Quality of Life Commission until July 2019 when she joined the city's Planning Commission during a once-in-a-generation Land Development Code rewrite, and is an inaugural member of Austin's first Independent Citizens Redistricting

Commission, which created single-member city council districts in 2014. Llanes Pulido was also part of the inaugural Community Strategy Team at the Department of Population Health at The University of Texas Dell Medical School, and is a 2019–2020 Fulcrum Fellow with the Center for Community Investment at the Lincoln Institute of Land Policy.

Tia Martinez, J.D., M.P.P., is the chief executive officer of ForwardChange and an independent consultant doing work on dismantling the school-to-prison pipeline and transforming life chances for boys and men of color. She has more than 25 years of experience creating social change in low-income communities and communities of color in the United States. Over the decades her work has spanned education reform, the HIV/AIDS epidemic, the war on drugs, homelessness, affordable housing, disconnected youth, and immigration. Prior to consulting, she was the chief equity officer at the Stupski Foundation where she designed a research and development effort focused on applying knowledge from psychology and neuroscience to help low-income students and students of color own and drive their learning and increase academic achievement. Martinez came to the foundation from the Warren Institute on Race, Ethnicity and Diversity at the University of California, Berkeley, School of Law, where she was the acting director of education, leading a policy unit focused on issues related to education reform, teacher effectiveness, and racial justice. Before joining the Warren Institute, she served as the strategic consultant to the Office for Civil Rights in the U.S. Department of Education, leading its strategic planning process and supporting rollout and implementation of the new strategy across 12 regional offices. Prior to working with the department, Martinez was a senior manager with the Bridgespan Group where she led engagements with large, national foundations and major civil rights groups. She has also been a senior fellow at the Hewlett Foundation, a policy analyst for the Corporation for Supportive Housing and the San Francisco Mayor's HIV Health Services Planning Council, and a street outreach worker. Martinez has B.A. in history from Harvard University, an M.P.P. from the University of California, Berkeley, Goldman School of Public Policy, and a J.D. from Stanford Law School.

Bobby Milstein, Ph.D., M.P.H.,† directs The Rippel Foundation's work on system strategy, is a member of Rippel's strategy and management team, and is a visiting scientist at the Massachusetts Institute of Technology Sloan School of Management. Milstein is a principal contributor to the ReThink Health initiative's Portfolio Design for Healthier Regions and Amplifying Stewardship Together projects. He also leads a suite of nationwide influence activities and coordinates ongoing development of the ReThink Health Dynamics Model, the Well-Being Portfolio Design

Calculator, and other simulation tools that let leaders play out the consequences of their scenarios for change. In 2018, Milstein and four co-authors wrote the official brief that defines "health and well-being" as the central focus for the Healthy People 2030 Framework for the United States. Before joining Rippel, Milstein spent 20 years planning and evaluating system-oriented initiatives at the Centers for Disease Control and Prevention (CDC), where he was the principal architect of CDC's framework for program evaluation. He received CDC's Honor Award for Excellence in Innovation, the Applications Award from the System Dynamics Society, and Article of the Year awards for papers published in *Health Affairs* and *Health Promotion Practice*. Milstein was once a documentary filmmaker whose work was used by PBS to spotlight challenges of racism on college campuses. He also contributed storylines for *The West Wing* on how to get beyond zero-sum thinking when setting health priorities. Milstein received his B.A. from the University of Michigan, his M.P.H. from Emory University, and his Ph.D. at Union Institute and University.

Laura Parajón, M.D., M.P.H., is the executive director of the Office of Community Health and an assistant professor in the Department of Family and Community Medicine at the University of New Mexico (UNM). She is the co-founder of the AMOS Health and Hope, a nonprofit organization that works with community health workers (CHWs) in remote areas of Nicaragua to improve health equity through health systems integration. As a family physician and a public health professional, Parajón is part of a team of CHWs, health professionals, and educators that uses community-based participatory research, a community empowerment approach, to work alongside communities, reducing child mortality up to 80 percent in remote rural areas of Nicaragua. Parajón received her M.P.H. from the UNM School of Public Health, her M.D. from the UNM School of Medicine, and her B.A. from Brown University.

Christine Petit, Ph.D., is an active leader in the Long Beach community and is the founding executive director of Long Beach Forward, whose purpose is to create a healthy Long Beach with low-income communities of color by building community knowledge, leadership, and power. She is also a co-founder of Long Beach Time Exchange—a time-banking community based on the premise that everyone has something to contribute to society. Petit serves on the Memorial Hospital Community Benefits Oversight Board and spent 2 years as the chair of the City of Long Beach's Board of Health and Human Services during her term on the board. With nearly 20 years of impact in nonprofits and community and labor organizing, Petit is an organizational founder and leader; a consultant to nonprofits, philanthropy, and government; and a certified life and leadership coach. She is also an advocate for children and families and is trained in trauma-informed nonviolent parenting, supporting children and families in the child welfare system, and mental health first aid. Petit earned her Ph.D. in sociology with emphasis in race and class inequality and social change. She taught sociology at California State University, Long Beach (CSULB), and was awarded Most Inspirational Professor by the CSULB Alumni Association in 2014.

Ai-jen Poo is the co-founder and the executive director of the National Domestic Workers Alliance (NDWA), a nonprofit organization working to bring quality work, dignity, and fairness to the growing number of workers who care and clean in homes, the majority of whom are immigrants and women of color. In 12 short years, with the help of more than 70 local affiliate organizations and chapters and more than 200,000 members, NDWA passed a Domestic Worker Bills of Rights in 9 states and the city of Seattle, and brought more than 2 million home care workers under minimum wage protections. In 2011, Poo launched Caring Across Generations to unite American families in a campaign to achieve bold solutions to the nation's crumbling care infrastructure. The campaign has catalyzed groundbreaking policy change in states, including the nation's first family caregiver benefit in Hawaii, and the first long-term care social insurance fund in Washington state. Poo is also a leading voice in the women's movement. In 2019, Poo co-founded SuperMajority, a new home for women's activism, training and mobilizing a multiracial, intergenerational community who will fight for gender equity together. She serves as a senior advisor to Care in Action, a nonprofit, nonpartisan group dedicated to fighting for a civic voice for millions of women of color, particularly domestic workers in the United States.

Poo has been recognized among *Fortune*'s 50 World's Greatest Leaders and *TIME Magazine*'s 100 Most Influential People in the World, and she has been the recipient of countless awards. She has made television appearances on *Nightline*, *MSNBC*, and *Morning Joe*, and her writing has been featured in *The New York Times*, *The Washington Post*, *TIME*, *Marie Claire*, *Glamour*, *Cosmopolitan*, and cnn.com among others. She has also been an influential voice in the #MeToo movement and attended the 2018 Golden Globe Awards with Meryl Streep as part of the launch of #TimesUp. Poo served as a member of the Bill & Melinda Gates Foundation–sponsored Partnership for Mobility from Poverty, and currently serves as a trustee of the Ford Foundation and a member of the Democratic National Committee. She has a B.A. from Columbia University and honorary doctorates from Smith College, the New School, and the City University of New York.

Lourdes Rodríguez, P.H., M.P.H.,*† is the senior program officer of St. David's Foundation. Prior to joining the foundation in 2020, Rodríguez served as an associate professor and the director of community-driven initiatives at the Dell Medical School at The University of Texas at Austin. Rodríguez also worked as a program officer at the New York State Health Foundation, and from 2004 to 2012, she co-directed the Urbanism and the Built Environment track in the Department of Sociomedical Sciences, Columbia University Mailman School of Public Health. As a public health practitioner, and in both academic and philanthropic roles, she collaborates, develops, and evaluates initiatives to improve health with people most affected by health inequities. Rodríguez has a P.H. from Columbia University, an M.P.H. from the University of Connecticut, and a B.S. in industrial biotechnology from the University of Puerto Rico at Mayagüez. She currently holds an appointment as an adjunct faculty with the UTHealth School of Public Health Austin Regional Campus.

Arvind Singhal, Ph.D., M.A.,* is the Samuel Shirley and Edna Holt Marston Endowed Professor of Communication and the director of the Social Justice Initiative at The University of Texas at El Paso. He is also appointed, since 2010, as the William J. Clinton Distinguished Fellow at the Clinton School of Public Service, Little Rock, Arkansas, and since 2015, Distinguished Professor 2, Faculty of Business Administration, Inland University of Applied Sciences, Norway. Singhal teaches and conducts research on the diffusion of innovations, the positive deviance approach, organizing for social change, the entertainment-education strategy, and liberating interactional structures. His outreach spans public health, education, human rights, poverty alleviation, sustainable development, civic participation, democracy and governance, and corporate citizenship. He is a co-author or editor of 14 books and has authored some 180 peer-reviewed essays.

Singhal's recent academic honors and appointments include Presidential Scholar, Mudra Institute of Communication Arts, India; President-Appointed Visiting Professor, Kumamoto (National) University, Japan; Fulbright Hays Scholar, Slovakia; Schomburg Distinguished Scholar, Ramapo College, New Jersey; Commerzbank Foundation Professor, Chemnitz University of Technology, Germany; Berkitt Williams Distinguished Lecturer, Ouachita Baptist University, Arkansas; and Raushni Memorial Deshpande Distinguished Lecturer, Lady Irwin College, University of Delhi, India. Singhal has served as an advisor to the World Bank, the Food and Agriculture Organization of the United Nations, the United Nations Children's Fund, the United Nations Development Programme, the Joint United Nations Programme on HIV and AIDS, the United Nations Population Fund, the U.S. Department of State, the

U.S. Agency for International Development, Family Health International, PATH, Save the Children, the BBC World Service Trust, the International Rice Research Institute, Voice for Humanity, and others. He has taught previously at The Ohio University, the University of Southern California, and the University of California, Los Angeles. He has visited and lectured in more than 90 countries across Asia, Africa, Latin America, Australia, Europe, and North America.

Daniel Sostaita, M.Th., is the pastor and the founder of Iglesia Cristiana Sin Fronteras (Without Frontiers Church) in Winston-Salem, North Carolina. In addition to pastoring his church, Sostaita also serves as a community connector for FaithHealth Ministries at the Wake Forest Baptist Hospital. Sostaita is deeply committed to the spiritual and physical wellness of his congregants and the local Latinx community. He has developed a Healthy Living Ministry at his church and provides a weekly free mobile health clinic in partnership with Wake Forest in the church's parking lot. Sostaita sits on the boards of the North Carolina Congress of Latino Organizations, the Hispanic League, and the Latino Network of the Cooperative Baptist Fellowship. In 2019, he obtained his life coaching license from METODOCC Christian Coaching and graduated as a prediabetes coach from the Diabetes Training and Technical Assistance Center at Emory University. Sostaita has a bachelor's degree in pastoral studies from Grace Seminary and an M.Th. from the International Baptist Theological Seminary of Cali, Colombia.

Paul Speer, Ph.D., is a professor and the chair of the Department of Human and Organizational Development at Peabody College at Vanderbilt University. Speer teaches community development theory, which examines the intersection of economics, politics, demographics, technology, and other forces shaping the urban form and the quality of interactions in these spaces. He also teaches community organizing, which explores expressions of agency by local actors on more macro-level processes, and the tools and methods for developing power to enhance action. Speer is currently involved in several community-based studies that draw on action research and participatory engagement with residents. He is working with a National Institute of Justice–funded study of youth safety and well-being and a Centers for Disease Control and Prevention–funded study of using media to alter community norms to reduce youth violence. Speer is studying community-organizing processes in a statewide effort with People Improving Communities through Organizing California and is working on a study of community-organizing efforts that are working to prevent the opioid crisis in Detroit, Cleveland, and Cincinnati. Speer currently serves on the editorial boards of the *Journal of Urban Affairs* and the *American Journal of Community Psychology*. Speer completed his Ph.D. in psychology at the University of Missouri–Kansas City and his B.S. in psychology at Baker University.

Meme Styles, M.P.A., is the founder and the president of MEASURE, a nonprofit social enterprise that provides free data support to Black- and Brown-led organizations, while charging white-led organizations the full rate of MEASURE's services to contribute to this anti-racist revenue model. Despite the odds and recognizing the need for increased information and data activism, MEASURE's accomplishments include the launch of the Travis County Girl Squad mentorship program; starting a data-activism course at Huston-Tillotson University; establishing an equity law in Pflugerville, Texas; advocating for the release of juveniles in response to COVID-19; led a study to help diversify philanthropy at the Austin Community Foundation; and advocated for the redistribution of funding from ineffective policing programs in exchange for evidence-based solutions. So far the organization has provided more than 1,300 free data support hours to Black- and Brown-led organizations. It is also responsible for strategic partnerships with The University of Texas, Texas Southern University, and more, with a goal of disrupting traditional research in exchange for Black- and Brown-led lived-experience protocols. Styles is not only the visionary behind MEASURE, but she is also an Austin Area Research Organization fellow; the past chair of Miss Juneteenth; the past chair of African TV5; the Austin 40 under 40 winner in 2019; and the recipient of the Austin Police Chief's Award of Excellence and the Austin Black Chamber's 2017 Community Leader of the Year award. Styles holds a B.S. in communications, an M.P.A., and is certified in performance measurement through The George Washington University College of Professional Studies.

Aditi Vaidya, M.P.H.,[*] is a senior program officer at the Robert Wood Johnson Foundation. Previously, Vaidya was a senior program officer for three sister foundations: the Solidago Foundation, the See Forward Fund, and the Frances Fund. Among her many initiatives with Solidago, Vaidya created Project Phoenix: Connecting Democracy, Economy, and Sustainability, a year-long cohort collective learning program for 40 participating foundations across health, democracy, economy, and environmental stability. Her prior work included serving as the campaign director for the East Bay Alliance for Sustainable Economy (EBASE), in Oakland, California. A community-based organization, EBASE unifies community, faith, and labor groups to stand with low-income workers and families. She also served as the program director for the Silicon Valley Toxics

Coalition, where she organized the first health and safety trainings for electronics workers. In this role, Vaidya coordinated campaigns to push California's high-tech industry to provide environmental and occupational health protections for communities and workers affected by the global supply chain. She has held other positions with the Jennifer Altman Foundation; the Southwest Network for Environmental and Economic Justice; the Center for Environmental Citizenship; and the League of Conservation Voters Education Fund. She was the board chair for the Asian Pacific Environmental Network; a former public health commissioner in Alameda County, California; a former member of the advisory boards of CorpWatch and the Labor Occupational Health Program of the University of California; a former steering committee member of the Labor Innovations for the 21st Century Fund; and a past co-chair of the Saguaro Fund of the Funding Exchange. Vaidya holds an M.P.H. in environmental and occupational health from Emory University and she earned her B.S. in environmental science and policy management from Bates College.

Bill J. Wright, Ph.D., is the director of the Center for Outcomes Research and Education at Providence Health and Services, Oregon and southwest Washington. Wright is a sociologist with a principal focus on survey design, and specializes in longitudinal research with low-income and vulnerable populations. His research focuses on the intersection of health policy, health systems design, and the social determinants of health. Wright has led numerous studies of low-income Oregonians, and he is a principal investigator on the Oregon Health Study, the first-ever randomized trial on the effects of health insurance. His other research has examined cost-sharing structures in Medicaid, the effect of continuity and churning in Medicaid, the effects of accountable care health reform on outcomes for people served by Medicaid, and the role of built and social environments as drivers of population health. Wright received his Ph.D. in sociology from South Dakota State University.

Hanh Cao Yu, Ph.D.,*† is the chief learning officer at The California Endowment (TCE) where she is responsible for learning, evaluation, and impact activities, and she ensures that local and state grantees, board, and staff understand the results and lessons of the foundation's investments in its 10-year Building Healthy Communities initiative. Yu led the effort to establish and implement the ongoing evaluation of the Move to End Violence. Prior to joining TCE, Yu served as the vice president; the director of the Youth, Education, and Philanthropy Division; and a member of the corporate senior management team at Social Policy Research Associates (SPR), where she oversaw much of the company's research and evaluation work in philanthropy. Yu has expertise in qualitative and quantitative research in the areas of women's philanthropy, leadership development, organizational effectiveness, policy evaluation, community organizing, and vulnerable populations. She has a wealth of experience in working with foundations to assess funding priorities, institutional change, program performance, and effective outcome measures. At SPR, Yu played a lead role in number of other projects, including the evaluation of TCE's Diversity in Health Evaluation Project, the evaluation of TCE's Health Exchange Academy, the TCE Diversity Audit, and the evaluation of the Kellogg Foundation's Capitalizing on Diversity Cross-Cutting Theme. Yu is the author of numerous publications and is a contributing author to *The Handbook on Leadership Development Evaluation*. She received her Ph.D. from Stanford University and B.S. from the University of Southern California.

C

Workshop Agenda

COMMUNITY POWER IN POPULATION HEALTH IMPROVEMENT

January 28–29, 2021

WORKSHOP OBJECTIVES

1. Understand the underpinnings of community-led initiatives.
2. Explore power (its dynamics, manifestations, and narratives) as it pertains to the agency needed for communities to articulate their health and well-being needs and act to address them.
3. Explore the approaches, elements, capacities, and ecosystems that support communities to lead their own efforts.
4. Explore the evidence base that links community power with systems of transformation and health equity outcomes.
5. Listen and learn from examples of community-led population health efforts in action.
6. Communicate insights from entities and sectors who are supporting community-led efforts.

THURSDAY, JANUARY 28, 2021

11:00 a.m. Welcome
Kirsten Bibbins-Domingo, Roundtable Co-Chair

11:05 a.m. Daring to Lead
Ai-jen Poo, National Domestic Workers Alliance
LaTosha Brown, Black Voters Matter Fund
Moderator: Tony Iton, The California Endowment

12:00 p.m. Community Power in the Context of Population Health
Richard Healey, Grassroots Policy Project
Jonathan Heller, Human Impact Partners
Moderator: Bobby Milstein, ReThink Health

1:00 p.m. Break

2:00 p.m. Community Power: Approaches and Models
Meme Styles, MEASURE
Roxanne Carrillo Garza, Healthy Richmond
Arvind Singhal, The University of Texas El Paso
Moderator: Lourdes Rodríguez, St. David's Foundation

3:00 p.m. From Vision to Action: Effective Ways to Support Grassroots Community Power Building
Hahrie Han, Agora Institute, Stavros Niarchos Foundation, Johns Hopkins University
Ethan Frey, Ford Foundation
Julie Fernandes, Rockefeller Family Foundation
Taj James, Full Spectrum Capital Partners
Mimi Ho, Movement Strategy Center
Moderator: Aditi Vaidya, Robert Wood Johnson Foundation

FRIDAY, JANUARY 29, 2021

11:00 a.m. Welcome Day 2
Ray Baxter, Roundtable Co-Chair

11:10 a.m. Community-Led Transformational Narratives
Rashida Ferdinand, Sankofa
Carmen Llanes Pulido, Go Austin/Vamos Austin
Daniel Sostaita, Iglesia Sin Fronteras

	Christine Petit, Building Healthy Communities Long Beach Michelle Carrillo, Del Norte and Adjacent Tribal Lands Moderators: Arvind Singhal, The University of Texas El Paso Gary Gunderson, Wake Forest Baptist Medical Center
1:00 p.m.	Break
2:00 p.m.	Amplifying the Empirical Base Linking Community Power and Health Equity Paul Speer, Vanderbilt University Tia Martinez, ForwardChange Bill Wright, Providence Health & Services Teresa Cutts, Wake Forest School of Medicine Laura Parajón, University of New Mexico Moderator: Hanh Cao Yu, The California Endowment
3:30 p.m.	Interactive Session The Basics of Power Building: Practicing the Community Organizer's One-to-One Meeting Method Ella Auchincloss, The Rippel Foundation
4:00 p.m.	Workshop Adjourns

D

Readings and Resources

Daring to Lead

- National Domestic Workers Alliance
  https://www.domesticworkers.org
- Black Voters Matter Fund
  https://blackvotersmatterfund.org
- Yes!, The Community Power Issue
  https://www.yesmagazine.org/issues/coronavirus-community-power
- Highlander Research and Education Center
  https://highlandercenter.org
- The Lead Local Collaborative, Leading Locally: A Community Power-Building Approach to Structural Change
  https://www.lead-local.org/findings
- Color of Change
  https://colorofchange.org

Community Power in the Context of Population Health

- Grassroots Policy Project
  https://grassrootspolicy.org
- Human Impact Partners
  https://humanimpact.org

- How Americans Can Reweave Our Fraying Social Fabric
https://www.minnpost.com/community-voices/2018/11/how-americans-can-reweave-our-fraying-social-fabric
- Thriving Together
https://thriving.us
- The Colorado Trust, Building and Bridging Power
https://www.coloradotrust.org/strategy/building-and-bridging-power
- Health Trust
https://healthtrust.org
- Connecting the Dots: Health Inequities, Power, and the Potential for Public Health's Transformational Role
https://humanimpact-hip.medium.com/connecting-the-dots-health-inequities-power-and-the-potential-for-public-healths-2b2f91eb3cba
- Power: The Most Fundamental Cause of Health Inequity? https://www.healthaffairs.org/do/10.1377/hblog20180129.731387/full/#new_tab
- If We Want to Advance Equity in Public Health Practice, We Must Address Race and Power
https://scienceblogs.com/thepumphandle/2016/01/07/if-we-want-to-advance-equity-in-public-health-practice-we-must-address-race-and-power
- National Academies of Sciences, Engineering, and Medicine, *Communities in Action: Pathways to Health Equity*
https://www.nap.edu/catalog/24624
- Story of Place: Community Power and Health Communities
https://dornsife.usc.edu/assets/sites/1411/docs/LEAD_LOCAL_Exec_Summary_091420_v1.pdf
- ReThink Health, Community Influence on Nonprofit Hospital Systems
https://www.rethinkhealth.org/wp-content/uploads/2021/01/RTH-CommunityInfluenceHosp_182021.pdf
- Call for Submissions: New Profit to Make $800,000 Investment in 8 Nonpartisan Democracy Organizations
https://www.newprofit.org/go/civic-lab-2021-loi/?utm_campaign=Announcements&utm_medium=email&_hsmi=105791117&_hsenc=p2ANqtz--Fk2lchz9B_vh5YZP7yPvDoVMEwwivqk-pIdt-BwZS-CwP_GzdtVVJ5Hq0r1uYaNB7mb4rUz3vQ1vKKpfKrrCTbalYde6ggwK5BlxA5J4gol-j7rU&utm_content=105791117&utm_source=hs_email
- The Social Ecology of Power in Participatory Health Research
https://journals.sagepub.com/doi/pdf/10.1177/1049732320979187

- Power, Control, Communities and Health Inequalities I: Theories, Concepts and Analytical Frameworks
  https://academic.oup.com/heapro/advance-article/doi/10.1093/heapro/daaa133/6056661
- The Three Faces of Power
  https://grassrootspolicy.org/wp-content/uploads/2018/05/GPP_34FacesOfPower.pdf

Community Power: Approaches and Models

- Manuel Pastor's 10 Key Elements for Movement Building
  https://bioneers.org/manuel-pastors-10-key-elements-movement-building-ztvz1802
- Supporting People Power to Achieve Health Equity for All Californians
  https://www.calendow.org/focus-area-list
- MEASURE
  https://www.measureaustin.org/home
- Richmond Community Foundation (RCF Connects)
  https://www.rcfconnects.org
- The Lead Local Collaborative, Exploring Community-Driven Change and the Power of Collective Action
  https://www.lead-local.org
- Positive Deviance Collaborative
  https://positivedeviance.org
- The Surprising Power of Liberating Structures: Simple Rules to Unleash a Culture of Innovation by Henri Lipmanowicz, Keith McCandless
  http://www.liberatingstructures.com/bookstore
- The University of Texas at El Paso, Social Justice Initiative
  https://www.utep.edu/liberalarts/sji/about/index.html
- National Latino Council on Alcohol and Tobacco Prevention, Take Action; Create Change: A Community Organizing Toolkit
  https://cdn.ymaws.com/www.wpha.org/resource/resmgr/health_&_racial_equity/lcat_take_action_create_chan.pdf
- By and for Residents: How Residents Built Power in North Richmond
  https://healthyrichmond.net/wp-content/uploads/2020/05/North-Richmond-Case-Study_07.30-FINAL.pdf
- Healthy Richmond Community Learning Plan and Evaluation Memo
  https://healthyrichmond.net/wp-content/uploads/2020/04/Healthy-Richmond-Interim-Evaluation-Memo_FINAL.pdf

Innovation in Measuring and Valuing Power for Community Action

- Ford Foundation
  https://www.fordfoundation.org
- Movement Strategy Center
  https://movementstrategy.org
- Agora Institute, Stavros Niarchos Foundation, Johns Hopkins University
  https://snfagora.jhu.edu
- Full Spectrum Capital Partners
  https://fullspectrumcapitalpartners.us
- The Lead Local Collaborative, Measuring Community Power for Health Equity
  https://www.lead-local.org/measuring-community-power
  Reports:
  1. *Reflections on Measuring Community Power*
  2. *Developing Community Power for Health Equity: A Landscape Analysis of Current Research and Theory*
  3. *A Research Agenda for Developing and Measuring Community Power for Health Equity*
- Robert Wood Foundation, Philanthropy Scan: How Funders View and Apply Power to Their Work
  https://anr.rwjf.org/templates/external/POWER_Philanthropy_Scan.pdf
- Walk With Us: Building Community Power and Connection for Health Equity
  https://www.rwjf.org/en/blog/2019/08/walk-with-us--building-community-power-and-connection-for-health-equity.html
- National Committee for Responsive Philanthropy, POWER MOVES: Your Essential Philanthropy Assessment Guide for Equity and Justice
  https://www.ncrp.org/initiatives/power-moves-philanthropy
- Building Community Power: A Philanthropic Strategy and End Goal
  https://www.ncrp.org/2018/07/building-community-power-a-philanthropic-strategy-and-an-end-goal.html

Community-Led Transformational Narratives

- Sankofa
  https://sankofanola.org
- Go Austin/Vamos Austin
  https://www.goaustinvamosaustin.org

APPENDIX D

- Faith Health NC, Radio Onda de Amor Connects Hispanic Community
  https://faithhealthnc.org/radio-onda-de-amor
- Building Healthy Communities—Long Breach
  http://www.bhclongbeach.org
- Building Healthy Communities—Del Norte County and Adjacent Tribal Lands
  http://www.bhcconnect.org/health-happens-here/bhcdnatl
- Groundwork USA
  https://groundworkusa.org
- Latino Community Foundation
  https://latinocf.org
- Pueblo y Salud, Inc.
  https://pys.org/about-pueblo-y-salud
- Group Health Foundation, Lessons Learned
  https://grouphealthfoundation.org/wp-content/uploads/2019/02/GHF_LessonsLearned_Updated.pdf

Amplifying the Empirical Base Linking Community Power and Health Equity

- AMOS Health & Hope
  https://www.amoshealth.org

The Basics of Power Building: Practicing the Community Organizer's One-to-One Meeting Method

- https://vimeo.com/rippelfoundation/powerbuilding

The Arts Supporting Community Power—Videos and Media

- Documentary: KCET, Power and Health
  https://www.kcet.org/shows/power-health/episodes/power-health
- Radio: Radio Onda de Amor
  https://www.radioondadeamor.com
- Let's Make Sweet Music Together
  https://medium.com/reimagining-the-civic-commons/lets-make-sweet-music-together-f19974f7228c
- TED Video: Ai-Jen Poo—The Work That Makes All Other Work Possible
  https://www.ted.com/talks/ai_jen_poo_the_work_that_makes_all_other_work_possible

- YouTube Video: What Is the Positive Deviance Approach? https://www.youtube.com/watch?v=0ULZWOm5ukg&feature=youtu.be
- YouTube Video: Positive Deviance Stories from Around the World https://www.youtube.com/watch?v=HhHHnP0UOZo&feature=youtu.be

Related Roundtable Publications

- *Supporting a Movement for Health and Health Equity: Lessons from Social Movements*
  https://www.nap.edu/catalog/18751
- *The Role and Potential of Communities in Population Health Improvement*
  https://www.nap.edu/catalog/18946
- *Exploring Equity in Multisector Community Partnerships*
  https://www.nap.edu/catalog/24786

The National Academy of Medicine

The National Academy of Medicine called on young leaders, ages 5–26, to use art to explore how the social determinants of health—factors in the environment where people are born, live, learn, work, play, worship, and age—play a role in shaping their lives and their communities. This is a list of some of the results. https://nam.edu/youngleaders/#/

- Imagine Belonging: https://nam.edu/visualizehealthequity/#/artwork/73
- The Community Cliff: https://nam.edu/youngleaders/#/artwork/156
- Health Equity Mural: https://nam.edu/visualizehealthequity/#/artwork/51
- Expecting: https://nam.edu/visualizehealthequity/#/artwork/68
- Chasing Sunshine: https://nam.edu/visualizehealthequity/#/artwork/20
- Neighborhood Community: https://nam.edu/visualizehealthequity/#/artwork/95
- Wishing Wall: https://nam.edu/visualizehealthequity/#/artwork/72
- Love Your Neighborhood: https://nam.edu/visualizehealthequity/#/artwork/41
- Burton Street Peace Garden: https://nam.edu/visualizehealthequity/#/artwork/106